AN AMERICAN YOGA:
THE KRIPALU STORY
By
James Abro

PRAISE FOR AN AMERICAN YOGA: THE KRIPALU STORY

James Abro's book, An American Yoga: The Kripalu Story, is a marvelous read. Abro's writing is meticulous, and at the same time, seamless and flowing. He synthesizes, with ease, the complex elements that gave way for the emergence of one of this generation's most well known yogic schools of thought. The Kripalu story comes alive as Abro explains the history and timeline of Amrit Desai's emergence from a remote, tiny village in India to renowned American yogi. He interweaves with ease and poignancy the story of Amrit Desai's guru, Swami Kripalvanandaji (Bapuji), and his dramatic evolution from probable suicide to sainthood. Abro's knowledge and comprehension of intricate yogic principles and his ability to transmit concisely and simply Kripalu's intriguing Shaivic lineage allows the reader to feel as if they have journeyed to ancient India and been let in on ancient yogic secrets. Amrit Desai, like many American gurus had a 'fall from grace' wherein many people were inadvertently impacted. Abro does a fine job sharing with the reader his understanding of the facts of this 'fall.' The book is not meant to be, nor is it, an exposé on Amrit Desai's wrongdoings but rather it is a vital historical reflection on how and why, in America, Kripalu came to be one of the most widespread practiced forms of yoga, one of the largest yoga ashrams, and one of the leading yogic educational centers of our time.

Zea (Tapasvini) Piver
*Former resident of
the Kripalu Ashram*

AN AMERICAN YOGA:

THE
KRIPALU
STORY

JAMES ABRO

AN AMERICAN YOGA: THE KRIPALU STORY
James Abro

Design
Gregg Hinlicky

Printed in the United States

First Edition
July 2011

Published by:
Aerodale Press
Post Office Box 1521
Toms River, NJ 08754
www.aerodalepress.com

ISBN 9781-4507-8624-9

CONTENTS

PROLOGUE

I t is my contention, having observed the Kripalu
phenomena for nearly three decades, that its
extraordinary success is due to something much
greater than the sum of its parts. And that the underlying
force behind the success of Kripalu – and what allowed it to
happen so quickly and seem effortless – is Grace.

Hence, my breaking down of the Kripalu Story into chapters
designating different aspects of this phenomena, from Grace Per-
ceived, to Grace Assigned, Husbanded, Skewed, Flourishing,
Squandered, Preserved, Restored, and Redeemed. Of course, Grace
does not unfold in such a linear way, but books do. So I've chosen
to break down the story of Kripalu this way for structural purposes,
knowing full well that the Grace needed for redemption in the 90s
was also readily available when Grace was being skewed in the
70s. The different forms Grace takes on in this story are constantly

intermingling, and I will let readers discern for themselves the apparent, and not so apparent, cause and effect relationship of each.

Grace is a phenomena recognized by most cultures throughout human history, though, as with most things, it's interpreted and experienced differently in the East and the West. In the West, Grace is referred to and interpreted mostly with allegory and symbolism, as a force descending from heaven and the gods, to earth and humans. The Greeks allegorized Grace as the divine attributes of Beauty, Charm and Joy rained down upon humankind whimsically via a pantheon of heroic and enigmatic gods and goddesses. And Christian theology symbolizes the descent of Grace to humanity in the form of a White Dove, the Holy Spirit.

In the East, Indian yogis have been working from the principle that "The Kingdom of God lies within," long before Christ proclaimed it. For them, God's Grace is a palpable force that exists within each human and is as universal and as necessary (and mysterious) for life as RNA and DNA. The purpose of yogic science is to foster an empirical understanding and practical application of Grace. The knowledge of the phenomenon of Grace that they have accrued over the ages is the essential, distinguishing, and monumental contribution of Indian yogic science to the amelioration of the human condition.

Western Christian theology places humankind in the position of having fallen from Original Grace through complicit interaction with Evil or the Devil, from which it can then be Redeemed through a Sacrifice of earthly desires and a Surrender to a Higher Power. This process can then be Sanctified by a Descent of the Holy Spirit into the Aspirant. Redemption, preceded by Falling, and followed by Atonement and Sanctification, are the key elements in this Western process of receiving Grace. Implicit in the Western schemata is that one must fall first before receiving Grace. Perhaps the most eloquent secular expression of this is the song, 'Amazing Grace', written by a slave-ship Captain in the middle of a life-threatening storm. God Gracefully saves him and his crew from death, and in turn he repents, amends his wretched ways and, in the process, writes a classic dirge of Atonement.

There is no such parallel in the Eastern formulation for receiving Grace. Absent is the need to sin, or fall, in order to be Sanctified. In fact, it's the opposite. In India, a spiritual mentor, or guru, selects from among his apprentices, or disciples, those whom he thinks are the most unsullied by life, solid in character, and sound in body and mind. Having spent a lifetime scientifically nurturing Grace, the mentor can, if he wishes, then pass on this knowledge through the teaching of practical disciplines, the reading of sacred scriptures and, distinctively, via nonverbal spiritual transmissions. It is through this process that yogic knowledge has been handed down from guru to disciple for more than 5,000 years.

The purpose in practicing yoga (I'm obviously not talking about performing postures at a health club) is to attain the ultimate State of Grace, or *Jivan Mukti*. In this exalted state, one unconditionally recognizes the Divine within, and without, and acts accordingly. Along the way to *Jivan Mukti*, adept yogis or gurus learn how to access the potential power of Grace, and share it incrementally, as needed, with their apprentices or disciples. This is the function of a guru: everything else, hoo-ha.

Western neuroscientists decades ago theorized (based on scientific study and anecdotal observation) that human beings function using only about one tenth of their brains' capabilities. Indian yogic scientists would concur and add that most human beings are also functioning with only about the same amount of their emotional, physical and psychic wherewithal. The antidote prescribed by yogis for this false anemic condition is the conscientious study and application of the disciplines of yoga, called *sadhana*, in order to achieve reunion with the true self, *Jivan Mukti*. ('Reunion' is needed to overcome negative cultural conditioning, not personal sinning.)

This brings to mind another song, dear to my heart having grown up Motown, which is Diana Ross's 'You Can't Hurry Love'. Well, one also cannot hurry *sadhana*, or *Jivan Mukti*. But try telling that to Westerners – and especially Americans – who are not renowned for their patience, or their willingness to wait on anything that can possibly, in any form, bring something good into their lives.

But rather than talk in general or analytic terms about the opposing and complimentary concepts and outlooks that characterize the relationship between Indian philosophy and American pragmatism, I prefer to offer AN AMERICAN YOGA: THE KRIPALU STORY. Because within this story, in microcosm, there is contained all of the profound cross-cultural alliances, betrayals, advances, back-flips, quests, misadventures and wonder that has defined the ongoing relationship between East and West.

"I do not understand the mysteries of grace – only that it meets us where we are, but does not leave us where it found us."

Anne Lamottt, Traveling Mercies

Dedicated to the Lakulish lineage
of yogis who brought
Kripalu Yoga to the world;
and to the many Americans, and others,
who helped refine and redefine
the delivery of that message.

CHAPTER 1

GRACE & ME

I first encountered Kripalu and Yogi Desai in 1980, a year after the Kripalu Fellowship opened a Holistic Health Center at a former corporate retreat they purchased in Summit Station, Pennsylvania. A national magazine, New Age Journal, which started up around the same time as the Kripalu Ashram, 1974, and whose niche was monitoring and supporting the trend toward holistic health and alternative forms of spirituality in America, asked me to go there and write a description of the facilities and services. They'd work my piece into a feature article they were writing about places for "alternative healthy vacation getaways".

I reported to them that the facilities were spartan. One slept, ate and attended programs in the same one large room. At night, in sleepingbags on the floor, and during the day, seated on the same bags folded up during programs and meals. Breakfast, lunch, and dinner were bland variations of rice and steamed vegetables. I also reported that the residential staff was welcoming, and eager to provide first-rate programs and services at very reasonable prices. I opined that if the Kripalu Holistic Health Center ever moved to a less remote location with better facilities, they could become a very popular destination among those seeking an alternative healthy holiday retreat. If not, their prices and programs would allow the Kripalu Retreat to remain a 'best kept secret' type of place among people who did not require standard amenities but who were actively seeking personal growth and a like-minded community for support.

(I squarely fell into the latter category then, as I still do. My most recent interaction with Yogi Desai was at a small yoga studio sandwiched between a deli and an immigrant social club just outside Center City, Philadelphia where Yogi Desai conducted a *satsanga* with as much gusto and integrity as he would have done, and has done, for a crowd of thousands. There were about twenty of us there with the sounds of urbania whistling through the room. In modern American parlance, Yogi Desai's got 'street cred'.)

A New Morning in America': Ronald Reagan, circa 1980

If you can, please try to recall 1980, which is now just about three decades behind us. Ronald Reagan was beginning his first term as president, swept into office on the wave of a feeling for returning America to its lost 'grass roots' values: meat, potatoes, and nothing to rock America's self-satisfied notion as the greatest nation on earth.

Enter The Kripalu Retreat, offering yoga, massage, acupuncture, chiropractics, homeopathy, herbalism, aromatherapy, psychic-readings, colonics, vegetarianism, astrology, chanting, dancing, and 'personal growth' programs. You name it.

Wow!

Looking back, as America tried vainly to tamp down a call for radical change brought on during the 60's, and return Americans to 'traditional values', The Kripalu Retreat and Ashram moved along blithely enticing its community and visitors to an even more fundamental return: to the primal atmospherics of the early days of our Universe when free-spirited divinely-inspired whirls of cosmic gases creatively formed something absolutely new and solid.

A new morning in America, indeed.

Back to Basics (if you will): 'Hara' Training

At the time I was available to go to the Kripalu Center for Holistic Health in 1980, they were offering a week-long intensive program called 'The Hara Training Program.' I'd never heard of a 'hara', but was game to find out, so I enrolled in the program.

It turned out that the *Hara* is a Japanese term for describing an area of the body that resides just below the navel and right above the pubic bone. The Japanese considered it to be one of the most important vital energy centers in the body, so they designed exercises to isolate and strengthen it. These exercises were essential in training samurai warriors and summa wrestlers. What I experienced there for six days was the following: a challenging, expertly run program supervised by Dr. Don Stapleton, a bright, youthful, agile and charismatic instructor. Dr. Stapleton would later become Director of Curriculum for The Kripalu Center when it moved to Lenox, Massachusetts. Following Yogi Desai's departure, Dr. Stapleton would take over as President of the Board of Directors of the Kripalu Center and guide it to a successful transition.

Like everything else at the Center, the Hara Program was designed to prepare the average person, and body, for one day possibly taking on the Herculean demands of practicing an in-depth form of yoga such as Kripalu Yoga.

Although some of the concepts and exercises were strange, difficult, and seemingly impossible, Dr. Stapleton instructed and demonstrated with such ease and good-nature that he made it enjoyable to try to keep up with him. We were also assured by him that this program had not been designed just for 'weak-haraed' guests/dilettantes like us, but that the entire Kripalu community was taking this training as well. And it was assuring to know that the community itself was practicing what it was preaching to us.

When an intensive weeklong program like this ended, it was customary, when Yogi Desai was available, for him to lead a group celebration *satsanga* and then take questions from those who participated in the program.

After six days of eating, sleeping and taking classes in one room, I was weary of being in the Center building, so I wandered out onto the grounds, which were surrounded by small run down post-mining-boon towns and unkempt family-owned farms. I'd been forewarned that the local populace looked upon the Center, its backpacking guests, yogis and yoga, like uninvited and unwanted in-laws. So I stayed on the property. It was a warm, early summer evening and as I walked, I closed my eyes so that I could better feel the effects of the week-long hara training program on me. I felt realigned (or perhaps aligned for the first time as an adult), stalwart, clearheaded, and effortlessly walking straight and supple. It was enjoyable to be in my body in this state.

I was so grateful to the staff and Center for helping me feel this way that it was with a good nature and lighthearted curiosity that I waited to see the community's guru. All week the staff had been priming us for experiencing him, who they referred to with affection and wide-eyed awe as Gurudev. I can safely say for the group I was in that many of us would have cut and run from such cultist-sounding promos if we thought we could have found a local, and friendly, alternative place to celebrate our new-found *haras*.

A path had been made for Yogi Desai from his residence to the Retreat. The stony path was strewn with flower petals, framed by lit candles, and lined with freshly showered, groomed residents dressed in Indian saris and dhotis, dresses and pantsuits. Most residents wore jeans and flannel during the day, so this sight was striking and appealing.

Yogi Desai suddenly appeared alone at the top of the path, raised by a small mound of earth, as though out of thin air. He was wearing a one-piece white tunic with gold embroidery, and sandals. I was twenty-six years old; Yogi Desai forty-eight. He appeared surprisingly youthful to me, and not as foreign-looking as I was expecting. With a thick wavy mane of black hair flowing down his back like a rock star, he looked very contemporary and approachable.

He moved forward fluidly, lifting his slender hands under his chin while bowing and nodding to each person along the path, including me, as I was easily drawn to the spectacle, and him.

When he looked at me, his eyes shimmered and appeared dilated. His smile was active, engaging, and contagious. When he smiled, you couldn't help smiling back. And when he looked into your eyes, it felt as though he was peering into you, or greeting and acknowledging something in you that he was more familiar with than you were. I felt myself smiling nonstop, and giddily, as though I'd just gotten high on something. My only previous experience of seeing anyone looking like Yogi Desai might have been someone who'd taken a dose of LSD and was having a very nice trip -- and from whom I was receiving a mild though pleasant 'contact high'. I learned later that neither the Kripalu community, or its guru, indulged or experimented with the cornucopia of recreational and 'mind-expanding' drugs readily available in America at this time.

I watched him go down the lane and I could see each face, like mine, light up as he passed. No words were exchanged, though I sensed that the heightened affectionate feelings flowing back and forth were in fact authentic, mutual and enriching.

I'd never experienced anything quite like this before so, naturally, I followed him and the others back into the Center. There, Yogi Desai gracefully assumed the lotus position on a plush red chair surrounded by flowers, a glass of water, and a harmonium (Indian hand organ). He paused, cleared his throat, and then began chanting in Sanskrit while vigorously playing the exotic-sounding acoustic percussive instrument. I'd only heard this kind of chanting before from the Beatle, George Harrison, at a benefit concert for Bangladesh at Madison Square Garden. Although that was also new and exotic to me at the time, in comparison to Yogi Desai's chanting it was plaintive and monotonous. Yogi Desai asserted the words of the chants, making them his own, while backing up his vocalizing with jazzy syncopations on the harmonium. The residents knew the chants, joined in, and soon they were dancing free-form all about the room. Some appeared to be in a trance. I noticed a few of my hara mates getting into it as well, though most non-residents, like me, were simply watching and listening in awe and wonder.

When the chanting and dancing wound down to silence and stillness, Yogi Desai took a sip of water and merrily asked if anyone had any questions. The part of my mind that formulated questions had either just left me, or gone into deep sleep. But out of the corner of my eyes, I noted a few of my *hara* training mates – a clutch of hearty and feisty Oklahoma cowgirls who had excelled in the program – striking their hands into the air. They wanted to know – heck, were demanding to find out -- why there were not any poor people, or minorities, present at the Retreat. I was living in an inner city at the time, and even though I was relieved and grateful to be out of the casually menacing environment for a week, I felt as though they had a point. Many American cities had been burned to cinders during the last decade and the demographics of the Retreat staff and guests reflected the polarization in America that I humbly felt helped instigate such disturbances. Yogi Desai candidly told them that he wasn't sure what they wanted him to do. So they went on to further ask why Kripalu did not offer scholarship programs, or some type of 'affirmative action' to help more people gain access "to something cool like this"?

Yogi Desai responded by saying that he didn't pick and choose who came to the Ashram, or the Retreat, and that those who were ready for it, or wanted it enough, found it.

With the names of more glorious sounding Deities than I could count still ringing in my head, incense wafting through my nostrils, and my gut feeling as solid as a samurai's, in that moment I actually felt as though I knew what it was. And more so, I smugly felt as though now I even had some of it.

Later, though, when I sobered up a bit, I would remark how awkward the exchange had been, as well as Yogi Desai's response.

But the article I was writing did not require me to report on anything more than the facilities and services. So I did not try to ask Yogi Desai any questions at *satsanga*, or privately, or report on my impression of him. For one thing, experiencing the Gurudev thing was new to me and completely beyond my ken. Additionally, it was apparent to me that Amrit Desai, the person, possessed innate qualities and attributes that would allow him to achieve his personal aims, whatever they were, with or without a community. And I very much wanted to see the Retreat, and its earnest and very likeable communal staff of residents, succeed.

Afterward, whenever I felt myself getting too far away from the easy sense of strength, well-being and clarity that I experienced at the Retreat, I'd return for a visit. Usually I'd pack a tent, camp on the property for a long weekend, and interact with guests and residents – some of whom in time became lasting and valued friends.

I would not experience Kripalu and Yogi Desai again until after the Kripalu Yoga Retreat moved from Pennsylvania to Massachusetts in 1984. There, as I predicted, it flourished as the Kripalu Center for Yoga and Holistic Health. Its staff became as highly regarded for their services and programs as Yogi Desai did for championing a new and distinctly Western in-the-world approach to yoga.

Shortly after they moved to Massachusetts, a friend, who was a resident of the original Kripalu Ashram, called urging me to come to the new Retreat in Massachusetts for an extended three-month stay. The retreat facilities in Pennsylvania were turning out to be a hard sell, and the Kripalu community was hard pressed to get their new facilities in Massachusetts up and running and bringing in revenues. They were looking for people to help out, voluntarily: the pay was room and board. What was more attractive to me at the time was an opportunity to be in a secure environment with a structured healthy lifestyle. My first novel had just been rejected, and a ten-year attempt at marriage was coming undone. I was living in Times Square during its pre-Disney *nadir*, and I was coming precariously close to mirroring the bleak and aimless trajectory of my surroundings.

It seemed unimaginable to me that I would leave New York City with so much unfinished business and go someplace to work for nothing. But within a month, my waning *hara*, or something, induced me to start moving in that direction. By the end of the month I had somehow managed to put my affairs in good enough order to allow me to trek up to Massachusetts and commit for a full three-month stint. Toward the end of my reinvigorating, though at times exhausting stay, someone told Yogi Desai that I worked as a professional writer and editor. Yogi Desai had been working on a book about Kripalu Yoga for several years, and his resident/disciples were on the look out for ways to support him in that endeavor.

Additionally, other pioneering East-West spiritual sojourners were putting out bestsellers at this time. The Kripalu community was leaning on Yogi Desai – in a good way -- to do the same. They were experiencing first-hand his knowledge and experience, and they wanted to help him to express it in words.

To this point, the Kripalu community had offered its best Ph. D's and former English teachers to work with him as his 'editors'. Anyone even remotely connected with the craft of putting words into print knows that that is not a winning formula for 'getting a book out', which is what the Kripalu community wanted most .

After reading a substantial body of his writing – every one of his public discourses was recorded and transcribed -- I recognized that the initial reaction I had to his dialectic with guests at the Retreat in Pennsylvania had been accurate. It was not the logic or clarity of Yogi Desai's spoken discourses that made you respond favorably to him and what he said, it was his sincerity, passion, charisma, plus the atmospherics. However delightful it was to hear Yogi Desai talk on the subject he dedicated his life to – Kripalu Yoga -- the words alone on paper did not match with the experience of hearing and seeing him deliver them.

Up until then, the writing and 'editing' process had been for him to select excerpts from his various discourses and then have someone cut and patch them verbatim into the chapters of a book. After we agreed that that wasn't working, I was able to get Yogi Desai to re-write his spoken discourses that I could then actually edit and work on with him. That helped him to produce Kripalu Yoga: Meditation in Motion, published by The Kripalu Yoga Fellowship in 1985.

While we were working on the book, I asked Yogi Desai what had prompted the Kripalu Fellowship to open its first Holistic Health Center in 1979. By this time, in its new location, the Kripalu

Center for Yoga and Health had become a multi-million dollar business by streamlining its original array of offerings to yoga classes and yoga teacher training, health services, and personal growth programs. It seemed to me that whoever first came up with the idea must have had incredible foresight and marketing acumen.

Yogi Desai looked at me genuinely surprised, and slightly bemused by my question and observation. Then he went on to explain that the primary reason they started up any kind of business was to allow residents to work from where they were living -- in order to facilitate their lifestyle and spiritual practices. Being of service to others, or *karma yoga,* was also a part of the overall Kripalu yogic regimen.

Yogi Desai is fond of writing and reciting aphorisms and he shared this one with me, "Company is stronger than will." He went on to explain that residents, especially new ones, needed the daily support of one another in order to maintain their new lifestyle and spiritual practices.

He then went on to further explain that the only requirements he had for any programs or services offered by the Health Center was that they be complementary and supportive of the practice of yoga. He pointed out that, in India, a serious student of yoga embarks on a rigorous regime of cleansing and purifying the body and mind (a mild example of such practices is called *neti,* which requires one to pour warm salty water through one nostril and out the other) that he felt were unsuitable for Westerners. (I agreed.) So if the Health Center could provide massage, saunas and supervised fasting to replace more austere ways one practiced cleansing and purifying in India, Yogi Desai was all for it.

I was also curious how the 'self-improvement programs', which had become the hallmark of the Kripalu Retreat, fit into a yoga regimen. One of the most popular programs, 'The Inner Quest Intensive,' required participants to spend a week or more quietly examining themselves -- how they ate, what they thought, what they said, and even how they walked. The purpose of these programs was evident to me, but how they complemented a practice of yoga was not. Like most people, I associated 'yoga' with doing the postures or *asanas*.

According to Yogi Desai, personal growth programs were complimentary to the more sublime and esoteric practices of yoga, such as repeating mantras and chanting devotional hymns, that were designed to help people break away from habitual subconscious negative patterns of thinking and acting in order to replace them with more conscious and positive ones. Additionally, programs designed to increase one's self-awareness and self-esteem were a way of preparing yogic practitioners for becoming more self-directed in practice and life -- one of the major innovative purposes of practicing Kripalu Yoga.

When we finished working on the book, I wrote an article about Kripalu Yoga for *Yoga Journal*. There were many new varieties of yoga inundating the American landscape, and Kripalu had yet to distinguish itself, with the public, from them. So I featured a pictorial layout of Dr. Don Stapleton, and other residents, executing Kripalu Yoga's signature 'posture flow'. The article and pictures helped to establish Kripalu Yoga as a distinctly new, modern and comprehensive way of engaging an indepth understanding and experience of yoga philosophy and practice, stressing intuition, creativity and self-directedness.

Kripalu had its book, plus an article, and I enjoyed not only an extended period of time to heal my personal wounds, but an opportunity to work and get to know the person credited with discovering and developing Kripalu Yoga. It also allowed me to see first-hand what it's like to be the person, as well as an icon, responsible for an entire community's expectations, hopes, fears, doubts, desires, fantasies and delusions. I was therefore not as surprised as many when the cultural pressure-cooker popped a decade later.

I traveled, completed another novel, and would not engage Kripalu or Yogi Desai again until a couple of years after Yogi Desai resigned as spiritual director of the Kripalu Center. I first returned to The Kripalu Center in Lenox to take a short weekend program that was being led by a friend. Everything there seemed as it had before, except for an absence of pictures of Yogi Desai and a feeling that the Kripalu Center was now more of a business than a community, which in fact it was. Residents who stayed were paid salaries and lived independently in nearby towns. Many new staff, with professional business and organizational skills, were hired.

The transformation from a spiritual community retreat, to a non-profit educational center and retrea,t had enabled The Kripalu Center to survive a near financial meltdown following Yogi Desai's departure.

The executive staff I spoke to during my visit were still very concerned about the public's perception of Kripalu in the aftermath of the imbroglio that took place between them and their guru. They estimated that about a third of their public 'softly' supported the move to remove Yogi Desai as spiritual director of Kripalu, another third couldn't understand what happened or why, and another third was belligerently opposed to the defrocking of 'their' guru. The Kripalu executives had their work cut out for them, though most seemed eager and excited about taking on the new challenges and opportunities before them. More than a few commented that it was now their time to be yogis, and to put into action, not just words, what they learned over the years by managing the Kripalu Center and practicing Kripalu Yoga.

To their credit, they did just that, in their own way. Although the Kripalu Center did look and feel more like a modern commercial health spa, Kripalu Yoga was still being taught, teachers trained, and the Center was bringing in many renowned authorities in health and spirituality to lead programs and seminars at the new Center. It was more corporate, but it was also more democratic and ecumenical. Though not intentionally, or even pleasantly, they had Americanized the practice and dissemination of yoga.

In the years I was traveling, my physical home in Times Square had been taken away as a result of a partnership between federal re.development funds and large corporations who assumed imminent domain over the few private non-commercial residences there. Times Square was now squeaky clean and thriving financially, without the tawdry 'businesses' it had formerly been infamous for. I resolved that if I could learn to go with the flow of that, and appreciate it despite my personal loss, I could also accommodate having my spiritual home become transformed and modernized. But it still felt odd to me, when it sank in, to know that Yogi Desai was no longer a part of the Kripalu Center. So the very next day after the program at the Kripalu Center ended, I drove to Sumneytown, Pennsylvania, where Yogi Desai and his family were.

If the Kripalu Center in Lenox was restructuring and reorganizing toward more contemporary and acceptable norms, than it appeared as though Yogi Amrit Desai and his small crew of loyalists were returning to their original free-wheeling ways. The plain austere dormitory that had been built to house residents from the original Kripalu Ashram – the Desai's family home -- was now painted brightly and full of noisy life. I could hear rock music and dialogue from movies, see young bearded men and floral dressed women just hanging out, and watch cats and children scurry in and out of screen doors. It reminded me pleasantly of the early days of the first Retreat, when Kripalu seemed more carnival-like.

It was fall, chilly, and Yogi Desai came out of the dormitory to greet me barefoot. He had just finished being the subject of an intensive four-hour *Rolfing* session. He appeared, at first glance, remarkably lighter and unburdened.

He welcomed me warmly and we sat across from one another at a picnic table. I could see then that he had aged markedly since the last time I saw him. His face was gaunt, and there were gray streaks in his thinner dark hair. He told me that the last couple of years had been the most difficult of his life. Mainly, he went on, as a result of being cut off so suddenly, dramatically and, ultimately, from the community of people he had lived and worked with his entire adult life.

He looked over at me sadly, and then an indefatigable sparkle and shimmer returned to his eyes as he told me, "I am so happy to just be free, to be myself again, and not the symbol and head of an *Ashram*."

I could feel that. It's how I knew him. Why we were sitting there at that moment. I did not come to him as a loyal 'disciple' – or as an investigative reporter, but as a concerned person, a friend.

Then he went on to tell me excitedly about seminars he would be giving soon in Belgium and Israel, and about the ongoing work he was doing at the Chopra Center in California.

When he got up to leave to take care of some business inside, I remained seated on the bench and watched as a swatch of listless pastel clouds descended slowly over a clump of gray hills on the horizon. I closed my eyes and breathed in. The air cooled, and the soft colors quelled within me. Delightedly, I breathed out and opened my eyes, not knowing where I would go next, or what I might do.

CHAPTER 2:

GRACE BESTOWED

I n February 2007, I traveled to Mumbai, India, in order to meet with Yogi Amrit Desai and a small group of people who were taking a 'lineage tour' of various places in India that are of seminal importance to the history of Kripalu Yoga. Kripalu's yogic pedigree traces its roots back to the second century CE, when an historical figure named Lord Lakulish founded the Pashupats sect of yoga, from which Kripalu Yoga is derived. Lord Lakulish is revered as an incarnation of Lord Shiva, and credited with systematically formalizing the earthly practice of yoga. Our itinerary included a trip to the temple in Kayavarohan, which is dedicated to Lord Shiva and houses an extraordinary likeness of the yogic body Lord Shiva appeared in as Lord Lakulish.

Our first destination would be a visit and stay at a temple under construction that was located outside a small village called Malav, located in the Gujarat District of southwestern India. One of the significances of the temple in Malav is that it was being built over the entombed remains of Shrii Kripalvanandji, Yogi Desai's guru and the namesake of Kripalu Yoga. It was widely felt in India, as well as among devoted yoga practitioners throughout the world, that Shrii Kripalvanandji in his lifetime achieved a rarified state of yoga mastery called *nirvana yoga* (absolute liberation), and following his death, or *mahasamadhi*, many viewed and experienced him as a saint possessing and dispensing eternal metaphysical attributes.

After a weekend in Mumbai to acclimate, we flew to the city of Baroda and then boarded a chartered bus that would take us to the village of Malav. Except for Yogi Desai and his son, Malay, none of the rest of us in the entourage were Indian, and only a few had previously been to India. Of the Westerners, I was the only one

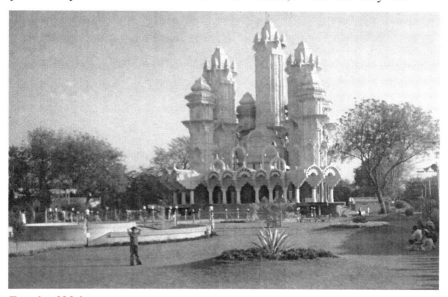

Temple of Malav

who knew Yogi Desai from before the end of his tenure as the
spiritual director of The Kripalu Center thirteen years earlier.

As most of us were encountering one another for the first time,
the atmosphere in the bus was informal, relaxed and chatty as
we eagerly exchanged stories about what brought each of us here.
After about an hour into the trip Yogi Desai, who was sitting in the
front of the bus, stood up and went into the cab to talk with the
driver. He came out smiling gleefully, and then announced that we
were going to be taking a little detour in order to visit the village
where he spent the first ten years of his life. Eyes twinkling, he
went on to tell us, "Those of you who only know me and how I
live in America are going to be very surprised to see where
and how I grew up."

Well, except for his son, that was all of us. Though in the course
of doing research for writing this book I'd looked through some of
Yogi Desai's archival materials and photos. So I knew that when
Amrit Desai was growing up in this small village called Pratappura
there were about 250 residents. Photos of the village, including
ones taken of Amrit Desai as a boy with his mother, father and
siblings, had to be at least six decades old.

I presumed that, as with most places in this day and age,
Pratappura would have changed dramatically over that amount of
time, and be rendered unrecognizable. I began to get my first
inclination that I might be wrong when the bus driver announced
that we were there, and simply pulled off onto the side of the highway to let us disembark. There were no signs on the highway
marking our arrival in Pratappura, nor was there a road from the
highway leading into the village.

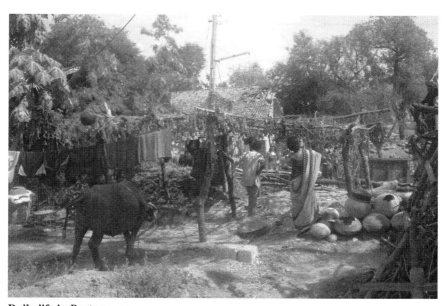

Daily life in Pratappura
much the same today as it was when Amrit Desai was growing up there

Our bus was modern and air-conditioned and the first thing we noticed as we walked off of the bus was a palpable wave of heat engulf us. I recalled that the average mean daily temperature in Gujarat was nearly one hundred degrees. I felt relieved that we'd come here in the 'cool' part of the year.

Our group variously walked, scuttled, and slid down a scree of rocks, pebbles, and fine gravel that safely raised the highway up and away from the surrounding landscape. (The predominant driving style in vast, overcrowded India is as fast as possible and with horn blaring.) Yogi Desai led us along a dirt path through brush into a clearing that was filled with flat plates and round bowls hardening in the sun on the ground. The plates and bowls were made from a mixture of clay and cow dung, and served as the chief export and source of income for the village.

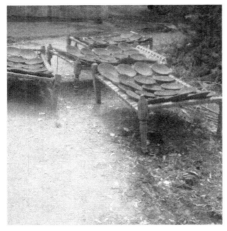

An elderly woman sitting in the shade of a lean-to made of stone with a tin roof, who appeared to be waiting patiently for the plates to dry and harden, greeted us with a mirthful grin. Yogi Desai returned her greeting by bowing his head, raising his hands in prayer position, and offering, "J'ai Bhagwan," a salutation that literally means, "I recognize and honor the divine in you".

Clay and dung plates drying in the sun

We each repeated the gesture as we passed, and the woman grew giddier and giddier, rocking and laughing in place.

We then entered the village – a variety of fifty or so small- and medium-sized makeshift shelters circumnavigated by an unpaved dirt pathway. Cows and oxen meandered freely. The present state of the village was not just similar to the pictures I'd seen from sixty years earlier, except for a few motor scooters, it was exactly the same.

Children ran out from their homes and schoolrooms and swarmed us. They yelped, giggled, danced, laughed and made us their playthings. I've traveled and lived before in places where people were 'deprived' of TV and other electronic distractions, so I was somewhat prepared for the onslaught of raw unfiltered energy. But the level of kinesis exuded by these children was something special. The girls, dressed in brightly colored pastel saris and with their faces painted and pierced, and the dark skinned boys wearing bright white school-uniform shirts and swirling around us like dervishes, made it feel as though we were being abducted by a colorful tribe of mystically charged mini-people.

Yogi Desai good-naturedly and patiently allowed them to do their thing, and then explained to them in Gujarati what it was he and we were doing there. He then told them with words and hand gestures that they could flank us quietly and follow us around on our tour of the village if they wanted. Most were too excited and restive to accept such an invitation and bolted, but several of them did as he asked, and that's how we proceeded into the village.

It was remarkable to me that a dozen or so camera carrying light skinned foreigners could walk into a self-contained hamlet like this unannounced, unexpected, and not receive a single suspicious or even circumspect glance. In fact, eye contact invariably triggered a mirthful grin or welcoming smile, as though there was a button within the villagers eyes that made their lips automatically soften and widen when you looked at them. The impromptu smiles and grins were more than welcoming; they were contagious and

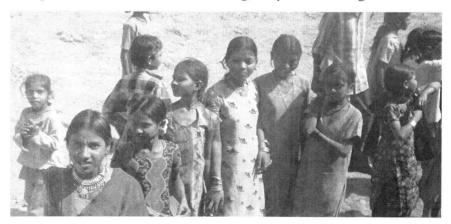

Children greeting us as we enter Pratappura

uplifting.

Immediately, our own circumspect feelings and logy pace picked up and became more spirited, liberated. Behind Yogi Desai and the Indian children, we nearly pranced into the center of the village.

The provisional-looking structures that served as permanent homes for the villagers did not provide much shelter from the elements, nor privacy. Windows and entranceways were not covered. In passing during daytime, one could look through from one end of the homes to the other, as well as see everything in between. Elderly people lying on cots in their homes fanned themselves with one hand and with the other waved out to us nonchalantly.

When we came to a stone structure with a tin roof and a small makeshift wooden porch attached to it that displayed various daily sundries, Yogi Desai told us that this is how his father had made a living for his family. "We rarely exchanged money. People would come in with what they had, trade it for flour or sugar, which we would then trade for milk, and so on." Then he looked up at a roll of shiny cardboard tags hanging from the top of the porch and flickering in the sunlight. "Only back then we didn't have lotteries."

In a book published by the Kripalu Yoga Fellowship in 1982, *The Life of Yogi Amrit Desai*, Yogi Desai described growing up in Pratappura in the following way: "Every morning I would awaken on my cot to the sound of my father's *hookah* (water-pipe) bubbling and gurgling as he waited for the family's bath water to heat. I could hear the crackle of the fire, while the sweet smell of the fire's smoke filled the room. My mother would grind flour at this time. There were two round stones, with a hole in the center into which she would constantly feed the grain. She would turn the upper stone by a handle to grind the grain into flour. While she was preparing the grain, she would sing *bhajans*, or devotional hymns. I would awaken to her sweet voice, the sound of the turning stones, and the songs of birds." [All the quotes in the remainder of this chapter, unless otherwise indicated, will be from *The Life of Yogi Amrit Desai.*]

Though he was a man of modest means, Yogi Desai's father, Chimanlal, was literate as well as a devout Hindu. In the evenings he would read to his wife and children stories from the *Mahabharata* or *Ramayana* -- lush, epic tales of the adventures, loves, misadventures, wars and fractious personal interactions among India's exotic pantheon of Gods, Goddesses, Demigods, and Androgens. "Our young imaginations were tremendous," Amrit recalled, "and the entire scene of every story would come alive in my mind more vividly than a movie. Every day, no matter what I was doing, I was always dreaming of where the story would go next. We were all eager to hear the continuation of these fantastic epics."

No matter how richly young Amrit Desai's imagination was being fertilized, I think it's safe to say that he could not have dreamt at the time that one day he'd live a parallel reality on another side of the world, and then return home for a show and tell with some of the people who were a part of that epic drama with him.

1942: HALOL, INDIA

When he was nine years old, Amrit Desai suffered a near-fatal bout of typhoid fever.

Following his recovery, the Desai family decided to leave

Pratappura. Sensing that their bright, imaginative, but shy and somewhat frail son might not be suitable for the types of occupations available to village-born Gujaratis – uneducated laborers or generational merchants -- the Desai family moved to a town where Amrit's grandparents lived and where he could continue his education. In the larger and more metropolitan Halol (population 17,000), there was a secondary school Amrit could attend, something that was not available in Pratappura or its vicinity.

Initially, Amrit found himself intimidated by the way of life and the vast number of people in Halol, which contained, after all, a population sixty times larger than that of Pratappura. He relates: "I had a disconnected feeling when we moved to Halol. I didn't understand what was going on around me. I had been a good student at Pratappura, and suddenly my grades fell. But once I caught up with my new environment, I became very sharp. What I lacked in social skills, I had gained ten-fold in living a very experiential life. From my upbringing, my mind was uncluttered and perceptive, and when I became comfortable in my new surroundings, my grades became excellent; not first in my class, because I preferred playing to studying, but always at the top level."

More attracted to active rather than academic pursuits, Amrit became the leader of a small group of boys who would get up early in the morning before school and exercise in the school gymnasium. One day during this formative period of his life, Amrit found a Gujarati translation of Dale Carnegie's *How to Win Friends and Influence People.* He not only read the book, but began practicing the principles and exercises for developing a positive attitude and optimistic outlook on life. For a young village boy trying to overcome shyness in the company of so many new strangers, this was a most welcome find. Decades later, when Amrit Desai returned to India with his family to attend his mother's funeral, one of his sons took the opportunity to rummage through his father's boyhood home in Halol. The son, Malay Desai, who had not only been born in America, but raised in a modern American *ashram* that doubled as a health spa, remarked that he could not believe first of all how meagerly and simply his father had lived in India. Then he reported that he was equally as surprised to find scores of notebooks filled with positive affirmations written by his father, noting that at that time no one was yet talking about affirmations, let alone writing them. Grinning, he concluded, "Especially in Halol."

Amrit Desai expressed it this way: "I wanted to work on myself and grow so much. I felt very inhibited in this desire and suffocated in my search for self-expansion. I wanted to read more, but books were scarce. I longed to travel, but there was no money. I wanted to build up my body, but there were no teachers. Our family couldn't afford highly nutritious food, or even a daily glass of milk. I wanted to grow spiritually, too, but my thirst for spiritual growth could not be satisfied by following rituals that my young heart could not understand. I needed a living religion, and a living person who personified the teachings, rather than just preaching about them."

In Halol there was a town square where actors, singers, and orators came to perform and speak publicly. One day a friend of Amrit's excitedly told him about a peripatetic teacher named Swami Chandra, who would be coming soon and reciting passages from the Bhagavad-Gita, the Hindu bible. Amrit was assured by his friend that this vibrant young man was not an academically or religiously trained preacher, but a former actor and poet from an upper class Brahmin family who had renounced worldly attachments and taken vows of renunciation in order to become a swami. A true living holy man. Intrigued that he might finally meet someone actually living the religious doctrines he'd been reading and hearing about all his life, Amrit made sure he was one of the first to get to the square that evening.

Amrit Desai recalled the first encounter vividly: "I went straightaway to the place where he was lecturing, and was immediately captivated. I knew that first day that he was my guru. When he spoke I had an inner knowing that everything I had been searching for in various ways could be found through him."

The fifteen-year-old Amrit Desai was too shy to approach the robust and outgoing swami, who was surrounded by an enthralled throng of adult townspeople. However, when Amrit found out that Swami Chandra was going to be staying in Halol for a fortnight in a loft over a barn that housed the town's sacred cows, he went to the loft every day after school to see if he could be of service to him. In Indian culture, it is a great honor to be allowed to be of any small practical aid to a holy man -- to quietly fetch him a glass of water or to fan him if he asks.

While Amrit had been exercising with his friends in the mornings, he came upon a chart depicting various basic yoga postures. Over time, he taught himself how to execute them. One day when Amrit was waiting outside the loft to catch a glimpse of the swami, a few of his friends came by and asked Amrit if he'd show them how to perform the yoga postures. Amrit obliged and, unbeknownst to him, Swami Chandra emerged from his residence and observed him instructing the other boys. The swami was so impressed with Amrit's enthusiasm, sincerity, and skill that the next day he invited Amrit in to show him a demonstration of the *sadhana*, or spiritual practices that Swami Chandra executed daily. It was the first time the swami allowed anyone to observe his *sadhana*.

Amrit Desai described the experience this way: "Bapuji (term of endearment for a spiritual father) invited me in, locked his door and entered into a deep state of meditation. After a short while, his body then began to move and flow in a state of automatic movement. The energy became so strong that his body was hurled across the room with tremendous force, dancing, weaving, moving in and out of complicated movements and *asanas* (yoga postures) as I watched in awe."

Prior to watching Swami Chandra perform *asanas* as part of his spiritual practices, Amrit Desai had not associated yoga with anything more than a form of physical exercise. The immediate effect of this seminal experience on Amrit was to ignite his curiosity about yoga, and deepen his commitment to practicing it. Swami Chandra noted this, and took a more active role in Amrit's personal and intellectual development. So much so, that three years later, when Amrit Desai turned eighteen and was eligible for marriage, Swami Chandra asked him to postpone his arranged marriage for five years in order to allow them to continue their yogic training together.

Amrit reacted to the request this way: "At that time I didn't understand why he was guiding me to wait so long, five whole years. But I trusted his insight for my life and approached my parents and told them what Bapuji asked me."

The following day, Amrit and his parents went to see Swami
Chandra. Amrit Desai's parents agreed with Swami Chandra's
request, seeing it as being in the best interest of their son's development. In turn, Swami Chandra assured them that Amrit was going
to reach a very high level of spiritual realization, and that the yogic
practice of *bramacharya* (sexual abstinence) at this juncture in his
life was going to aid him greatly toward that accomplishment.

During this intensive period of training with Swami Chandra,
Amrit noted: "As I increased my practices and strengthened my
observance of *bramacharya*, my energies became extremely
focused and alive."

There are not any moral or quasi-religious underpinnings to the
practice of *bramacharya* during specific stages of yoga. And there
is more to it than just not acting or reacting to sexual impulses. The
discipline involves a conscious and very difficult sublimation,
assimilation and internalization of sexual energy. While practicing
this discipline, Amrit Desai noticed that his creativity became
acutely enhanced and his artistic perspectives increasingly lucid. It
was during this period that Amrit got his first job as an artist, painting marquees for the town's movie theater.

After completing his training with Swami Chandra, and
graduating high school, Amrit Desai made a move that astonished
everyone. He enlisted in the Indian Air Force . When I asked him
about that, his eyes sparkled mischievously: "I wanted to do the
most amazing, outrageous thing, something that no one in my town
would have thought of doing. To travel one thousand miles away
and join the Air Force was unheard of in our little town. Plus, I
wanted to learn how to fly!"

Amrit Desai initially did well in the Air Force. Though when they informed him that he was being trained to be a gunner, not a flyer, he purposely began performing his duties inadequately until they discharged him from service.

Afterward, he returned to Halol, took a job teaching art at the local high school, and at the age of twenty-three married the young woman he was betrothed to, Urmilla. A few years later, they had their first child, a son they named Pragnesh. Amrit Desai had a respectable job, a wife, and a healthy child. This would have been a very comfortable and accomplished life for a typical young man in Gujarat.

Characteristically, however, Amrit Desai did not find typical accomplishments adequate, nor the comfortable engaging. During his brief stay in the Air Force, for the first time in his life, Amrit Desai encountered people who had traveled outside of India. The ones he met who had been to the United States spoke excitedly and enticingly about a culture that was uniquely dynamic, open, prosperous and innovative. That was all that a bright young man looking for a way to expand his horizons needed to hear.

After deciding that he wanted to go to America, Amrit Desai consulted with his village elders -- including palm readers and astrologers -- to see if there were any favorable signs aligned with his unconventional plans. They knew that the bright and talented young Gujarati man was not only asking for their approval to leave the sacred womb of Mother India, but also a wife, a son, and a job, in order to go to a strange and exotic place that called its native population, of all things, Indians. And Lord knows what happened to *them*.

Predictably, the soothsayers divined no favorable signs. Undaunted, Amrit then went to see Swami Chandra, looking for a telltale from him that he should follow his instincts and follow through with his daring plans. Amrit Desai remembered the day this way: "He (Swami Chandra) was speaking at a festival. There were so many people there that I couldn't find any place close to him. So I sat far away and started to silently pray from my own heart, asking for his guidance: 'Bapuji, if you want me to go to America, please show me in some way.'

"Immediately, I saw Bapuji look through the crowd right at me, and from a distance he gestured with his hand for me to bring him a glass of water. There were many people nearer him to serve him, but he pointedly asked me to do this. In this way, I received my affirmation, and the blessing for my trip to America."

CHAPTER 3

GRACE MANIFESTS

I n Indian custom, an overcast, dreary day is seen as
auspicious, marking a favorable time to make a change in
one's life, and especially so if it involves traveling.

It therefore must have been a great relief – after
receiving dour predictions from the soothsayers, and with
only six hundred dollars in his pockets -- for the twenty-eight-year-
old Amrit Desai to disembark onto the tarmac in Philadelphia,
Pennsylvania on one outstandingly lackluster, rainy day in the middle of winter, 1960.

When Amrit Desai asked his bus driver to take him to Pine
Street in Philadelphia to meet with his one and only contact in
America – a friend of a friend staying at The International House --
the driver misunderstood his Gujarati accent and delivered him to
Vine Street. Amrit Desai then walked across a cold and blustery
Philadelphia dressed only in a light summer suit and new leather

shoes. When he finally reached his destination, he was to learn that his total financial resources – the six hundred dollars he was carrying -- was not enough even to pay for a semester's tuition at the Philadelphia School of Fine Arts. Additionally, he found out that his student visa prohibited him from working full-time, while his wife and child waited to join him in America as soon as he could afford to send for them.

He learned how to apply for and receive a student loan and then, while he waited on a hardship claim to his visa status, he found a non-paying job washing dishes in the college cafeteria in exchange for lunch. For several months it was the only daily meal he ate. When immigration finally issued a work permit to him, he took a full-time night-shift job at a paper bag manufacturing company for $1.50 an hour.

The typical day for Amrit Desai at this time was to take classes in the morning, work in the cafeteria during lunch, and then take a bus to his job at night. After work, in order to save money, he would walk home through Philadelphia's rough Southside.

As Amrit Desai went about his simple nightly tasks of assembling and packing paper bags, his mostly white co-workers became suspicious of his dark-skinned appearance, and put off by his quiet self-contained manner. They took to teasing him, and when they tried to entice him to go out with them after work for a 'good time', Amrit Desai would politely decline and quietly slip away.

His remarks about those times reveal his thoughts and feelings as well as his assessment of the influences that allowed him to remain focused on his goals despite the obstacles and distractions. "When I came to America, in your Western way of looking at it, I met with anything but success. I received total rejection at first from every angle. But strangely enough, I never felt rejected. There was no time for meditation or yoga. My lifestyle was a yoga: to be happy under all circumstances and to accept all that was adverse. To take life as it is: there is no yoga higher than that, and that level of acceptance is the result of practicing yoga." (*The Life of Yogi Amrit Desai,* The Kripalu Yoga Fellowship, 1982.)

That statement reflects an understanding of the tangible worldly benefits of yoga that will allow Amrit Desai to experientially trail-blaze a new and modern approach to the practice that will in time become so popular among Westerners. Amrit Desai is discovering, in his own way, that yoga is not something that has to be done while secluded in an *ashram* or temple exclusively for the purpose of spiritual development. In fact, when the practical and spiritual applications of yoga are combined, the benefits can then be enhanced, not compromised by life's experiences -- even while working in a paper bag factory.

It is not philosophy, or a set of lofty ideals that animate Amrit Desai's practice and exploration of yoga. It is the immediate benefits he receives, even in difficult circumstances, that brand it into him viscerally, and eventually makes it something he can't help but want to learn more about, and share with others.

Art or Yoga?

As a result of working full-time while attending college and living stoically, after a year-and-a-half Amrit Desai was able to bring his wife, Urmilla, son, Pragnesh, and brother, Shanti, to America.

By the time he graduated from the Philadelphia School of Fine

Arts in 1964 with a Bachelors Degree, he and Urmilla had brought a second child into their family, another son they named Malay.

During the next three years, Amrit Desai worked at several professional positions with commercial design and textile firms, while at the same time moving forward with a very promising independent career as an artistic painter. As an artist, he was garnering praise and recognition for renderings of traditional Indian motifs with modern Western painting styles. Desai's paintings were extraordinarily well executed and at the same time favorably aligned with America's sub-cultural tilt toward the Eastern, mystical and exotic. Savvy art dealers were taking notice. A year out of college and Amrit Desai's artwork was appearing at galleries in Philadelphia and New York City, producing sales to a growing number of collectors.

Even before graduating college, though, an event took place that greatly influenced Amrit Desai's destiny. While he was living at a dormitory for foreign-exchange students in Philadelphia, he was selected to represent India in a program called "International Day". He participated by demonstrating a few simple yoga postures, playing traditional Indian music on the flute, and offering a brief lecture on the basic principles of Indian spiritual philosophy and how they relate to yoga.

This was at a time when few Americans had seen yoga postures performed, nor knew that this strange and difficult looking form of exercise was part of a five-thousand-year-old tradition of spiritual practices. Add in the entrancing flute music, the earnestness and attractiveness of the presenter, and Amrit Desai found himself speaking publicly for the first time in his life, standing before an enrapt audience. On that day in 1962, Amrit Desai began to suspect that the main theater for his activities in America might not be as an artist, but as a personal emissary of Indian culture and spiritualism.

Invitations followed to speak at conferences and festivals, and soon Amrit Desai was talking and appearing on local radio and television stations. One of these television appearances took place on the Philadelphia-based Mike Douglas show, one of the first TV talk shows to syndicate nationally. Mr. Douglas became so successful in this new medium in part because he knew that talking was not enough to hold his viewers' attention. Intuiting on this day that he might be losing his audience while talking with Amrit Desai about yoga, Mr. Douglas – with the awestruck facial mannerisms of a carnival barker -- informed his audience that he'd heard yogis could lower their blood pressures at will. He then turned and challenged Amrit Desai, impromptu, to allow a blood pressure reading of him at that moment, and then again following the next commercial break, which was less than a minute away.

I've heard Yogi Desai tell this story at various venues over the years, and this is how it goes: "I wasn't sure what it was he was asking me to do, but I was a guest on his show so of course I thought I should try to go along with what he was doing. So I allowed them to put the apparatus on one of my arms in order to take a blood-pressure reading. Mr. Douglas called the numbers out to the television audience before the show paused for a commercial. I didn't do anything special during the break other than take a sip of water. When the show came back on the air, an assistant to Mr. Douglas took another reading and then Mr. Douglas shouted the numbers out to his audience and everyone clapped and cheered. I was so relieved that all I could think of was, 'Thank God'."

Demand for yoga classes arose from this kind of public exposure, though Amrit Desai still needed to continue working full-time as a commercial designer in order to provide for himself and his family. He found himself once again at a crossroads in life. He could either maintain a two-pronged career in art that was providing his family with a substantial and secure income, and him with personal recognition; or he could risk that security, and the lure of fame and possible fortune, in order to embark on teaching a discipline that was still very new to the West.

Amrit Desai made his decision to choose teaching yoga over making art because he felt that his early indoctrination into yoga is what allowed him to be successful in life so far. So why not apply yoga to teaching yoga, despite the difficulties?

When I asked Yogi Desai about his decision he characteristically put it more succinctly: "I chose the bigger canvas."

In 1966, Amrit Desai formally punctuated his decision to dedicate his life to teaching yoga by founding The Yoga Society of Pennsylvania. In that same year, he also traveled back to India for his first visit since leaving.

The Roots of Kripalu Yoga & The Temple of Kayavarohan

Naturally, one of the first persons Amrit Desai wanted to see and tell about his decision to devote his life to teaching yoga was Swami Chandra. When the thirty-four-year-old Amrit Desai arrived back in India brimming with excitement, optimism and anticipation about his decision to teach yoga in America, Swami Chandra was temporarily ensconced in an *ashram* in Mumbai (Bombay) while he awaited the completion of the restoration of a temple in the village of Kayavarohan. A few years earlier, Swami Chandra's guru had cryptically informed him that he, Chandra, was going to restore an ancient 3,000 year-old sacred temple that had been destroyed a millennia ago.

Swami Chandra had no idea what temple his guru had in mind, or how in the world he -- a penniless monk -- was going to go about accomplishing this task. But shortly after the instructions from his guru – who appeared only to him, intermittently, in an ethereal body – Chandra was invited to speak at a religious celebration in the town of Kayavarohan. Kayavarohan had been established about three thousand years ago and was recognized as the birthplace of Brahmin culture. As noted earlier, it was also the place where Lord Lakulish, believed to be the 28th incarnation of Lord Shiva, founded the Pashupats sect of Tantra Yoga in the first half of the second century CE. Brahmin culture and Tantra Yoga combined to usher in a golden age of social, architectural and scientific achievement in India, along with producing what is perhaps the finest body of spiritual literature and erotic art the world has seen to date. Then, in 1025 CE, Moslems razed the town of Kayavarohan, intentionally destroying its temples, erotic art and Hindu iconography.

After speaking at the festival, Swami Chandra visited a dilapidated temple on the outskirts of the town of Kayavarohan. There, he was astonished to see that on the main altar of this temple there was a massive black stone meteorite with the body of a yogi merged into it. The cylinder had been so large and dense that the Moslems couldn't destroy it, so they buried it. After nearly a century – in May of 1866 -- it was found, unearthed and moved back into the temple.

Swami Chandra immediately recognized that the yogi who had merged into the symbolic stone *linga*, or phallus, was *his* mysterious guru and that the temple he was going to restore was the Temple of Kayavarohan. (In Sanskrit, *kaya* means body, and *varohan* to descend. Kayavarohan is literally the place where Shiva descends or incarnates into the earth body. Being the male principle of Divinity, Shiva is often represented in earthly form by a *linga*.) Swami Chandra was humbled and overwhelmed to realize that Lord Shiva – one of the three main Hindu deities, along with Shakti and Brahman -- had incarnated in the ethereal form of Lord Lakulish in order to personally initiate and mentor him. When Chandra meditated before the icon of his guru and asked for guidance on how to undertake the formidable task of restoring the Temple, he received: *'Our chosen son, you have only to act as an instrument of the divine will. The task will take care of itself.'* [*Light from Guru to Disciple*, Rajarshi Muni, The Kripalu Ashram, Sumneytown, Pa., 1974.]

Later in the book, I will detail how Swami Chandra becomes Shrii Kripalvanandji and continues his yoga *sadhana* in America. For now, though, let us continue with an account of the auspicious reunion that took place between *Bapuji* and Amrit Desai in 1966.

Swami Chandra recalled the visit to India by Amrit Desai this way: "When I was in Bombay, Amrit returned from the United States. We met each other with feelings of deep affection, and he told me about his activities of yoga. During the intermediary years,

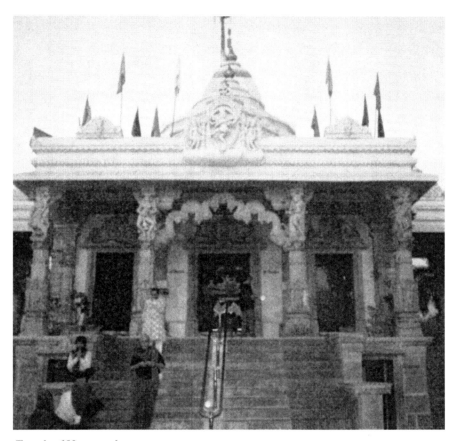

Temple of Kayavarohan

he had read many volumes on *Jnana Yoga* (Yoga of Knowledge),
Bhakti Yoga (Yoga of Devotion), and related subjects. Knowing
about his activities and his mentally inspired condition, my heart
leapt with great joy. He was initiated by me at Biwanda in the
Thana District near Bombay. He then stayed with me for about a
fortnight, while I taught him some techniques of yoga and gave
him some knowledge of the *Shastras*."

The *Shastras* are Indian scriptures outlining ways to the
realization of undistorted reality, or truth. Passing on esoteric

techniques for practicing and experiencing yoga, along with an intellectual blueprint for understanding something as elusive as truth, is the Indian equivalent of an American scientist passing on esoteric mathematical formulae, experimental techniques, and study habits to a young protégé trying to get a grip on quantum mechanics. In both cases, a teacher would not bother passing on the knowledge and experience if they did not think the student could understand and apply it.

Amrit Desai described their meeting as follows:

"Sometimes beloved Bapuji would ask me to read from the manuscript of his book, *Asanas and Mudras*. I often looked up as I read. Bapuji's eyes showered love on me, and I caught the glimpse of Divine light emanating from his eyes. I have no words to explain these experiences. Those eyes reflected the Divinity and love that he was communicating at all times. You have to see such a profound spiritual love in such a saint's eyes only once to remember it for the rest of your life. I call it sheer blessing to be fortunate enough to have had such heartstirring and moving moments with my Guruji."

The initiation, or *diksha*, formalized Amrit Desai's relationship to Swami Chandra and the Pashupats lineage of Tantra Yoga dating back thousands of years to its founder, Lord Lakulish. The equivalent to *diksha* in the early stages of Christianity would have been the spiritual initiation rites of Baptism and Confirmation. "Only the Transfigured One imparts the spirit to the community." (John 20:22.) But as the modern Church became centralized around a Pope, the practice of occultist transmissions through 'transfigured' members of the Christian community (such as John the Baptist and

Saint Francis) did not carry on. The current Evangelical movement
in Christianity seems to be attempting to revive it.

In India, it remains the essential way in which esoteric yogic
knowledge, grace and wisdom is passed on from guru to disciple.

In a letter to Amrit Desai, Swami Chandra elaborated in more
detail about what he felt took place during their reunion in 1966:
"So soon in your life, you are so centered and set in your goal of
yoga. Your experience is so much like that of many great souls of
the past. This I call the grace of God. This same grace is the divine
guidance behind me now, giving you these deep and hidden teachings
of yoga. "I am giving you what I have not given to anyone so far. I
want you to keep these teachings secret, even from your dearest

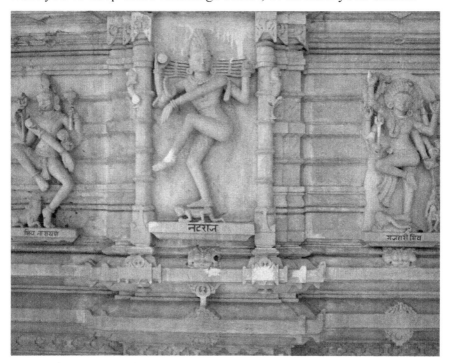

Temple of Kayavarohan facade

friend. You will understand their true meaning and value when you tread the path of yoga. These teachings will truly fulfill the purpose of your *sadhana*. "I pray that God may bring you this truth soon."

His remarks vividly underscore the sublime nature of how teaching and sharing is done in the yogic tradition. The guru transmits advanced knowledge he has received from his guru, and has experienced on his own, to an aspiring disciple who, if they stay on the path of yogic self-realization (self-realization and god-realization are synonymous in yogic epistemology) gain it on their own in their own time.

In following chapters, I will describe some of the profoundly mystifying, practical and bewildering ways in which this peculiarly Indian form of Grace manifested itself in America, and how it continues to do so.

CHAPTER 4:

GRACE DEVINES

The 'discovery' of a New Yoga in America

When Amrit Desai returned to the United States, The Yoga Society of Pennsylvania was expanding at a phenomenal pace. There were now more than one hundred classes taking place weekly, with over a thousand students a month.

Even today, with yoga assimilated into the standard American fitness curriculum, this many weekly classes and students would be outstanding. Additionally, in 1966 health clubs offering yoga and independent studios featuring an array of eclectic alternative health services and practices featuring yoga were not yet part of the American cultural landscape. The extraordinary growth of the Yoga Society was due almost exclusively to Amrit Desai's ability to personally recruit students. What he had going for him were attributes any Madison Avenue public relations firm at the time wished they could have bottled and sold: a handsome young man with a wholesome enthusiasm for his mission, charisma, a naturally flexible physique, and clean-cut appearance.

When Amrit Desai lectured about yoga he showed up in a suit and tie, and when he demonstrated even the most challenging yoga postures he did it with such ease and grace that it disarmed anyone's fears of this exotic new form of 'exercise'.

The increased demand for classes and instruction also created a need for Amrit Desai to begin teaching his students to lead yoga classes, as well as train some to do clerical and administrative work. As his yoga students began taking more responsibility for the running of the Yoga Society's operation, Amrit Desai felt it was important to begin introducing his student-cohorts to deeper aspects of the practice of yoga.

Even though teaching yoga was now, by choice, Amrit Desai's career, and the main source of his family's income, Amrit Desai did not want the Yoga Society to become just another business with its main focus on more and more classes and income. By focusing the attention of the Yoga Society's members on their practice of yoga, and letting the business take care of itself, a symbiotic relationship developed between the practice of yoga and the running of a cooperative business enterprise. A correlation that would not only, in time, characterize and distinguish the Kripalu community and enterprise, but pay dividends beyond what anyone then could have anticipated.

Amrit Desai's remarks about those times reveal how, for him, it was always the in-depth practice of yoga that needed to be primary; as well as how, in the beginning, it was not easy for him to assert that: "When I was a yoga teacher, for a long time I was afraid to

chant *Om* in my classes. I would justify this fear by telling myself,
'I don't want to do anything to disturb my students' faith in their
own religion.' After I returned from my first trip back to India in
1966, my heart was so open from Bapuji's presence that I sponta-
neously began to chant Om as part of my classes. "Bapuji then
wrote to me, 'You must do *Arti.*' (*Arti* is a ceremony during which
practitioners light candles and chant devotional hymns, symboli-
cally acknowledging and offering reverence for the Divine light
harboring in everyone.) I had been reluctant to do *Arti* since it was
quite unknown to Westerners, but I didn't hesitate a moment when
Bapuji asked me to do it. My fears vanished because I knew he
was guiding me in the best direction." (*The Life of Yogi Amrit
Desai*, Kripalu Yoga Fellowship, 1982.)

There are two very important insights into the guru-disciple
relationship and the practice of yoga to be gleaned from this quote.
One, is that the guru-disciple relationship is not at all similar to the
teacher-student dynamic experienced in the West. In the West, one
goes through life learning different skills from different teachers
over a lifetime; we don't select one person whom we unequivocally
accept to be our guide for life. Secondly, Swami Chandra is asking
Amrit Desai to let his students know upfront, through this simple
ritual, that yoga is essentially a spiritual practice.

As Amrit Desai steadily goes deeper into his understanding and
practice of yoga, his students – in the same way he had done with
Swami Chandra – begin to see him as a role model and guide, and
look for ways to be of service and support to him. Amrit Desai's
leap of faith – to leave behind a relatively secure career in order to
follow his heart and intuition – is followed by a leap of their own.

No one at this time was joining the Yoga Society because they felt it was a good career move. Like Amrit Desai, many of the members of the Yoga Society were recent college graduates who had not planned on using their education and training in order to join an alternative spiritual community and teach yoga. And no one at this time, not even a Cassandra, could have envisioned America's sudden tack toward health and fitness that would so favorably parallel the fortune and success of the Kripalu community.

As the community faithfully studied and practiced yoga and became more and more pregnant with potential, so did the Desai family, literally. In March of 1968, a baby girl they named Kamini was born into the Desai family.

The Cats Get Out of Their Bags & Will Do What?

In 1969, Amrit Desai received a formal invitation from Swami Chandra to return to India in order to stay for a five-month period of intensive *sadhana*. (At this level, sadhana is an all-encompassing embrace of the multi-faceted aspects of yogic spiritual training, including esoteric breathing exercises, meditation, scripture study, chanting, prayer and other practices that I will describe as we go on.)

In the three years since Amrit Desai last saw him, in recognition of his dedicated study and advanced application of *Kundalini* Yoga, Swami Chandra was offered an *ashram* to head in Malav, India, where he'd be addressed formally from then on as Shrii Kripalvanandji, the saintly, exulted and compassionate one. This is how Amrit Desai described his extended period of time with Shrii Kripalvanandji:

"I sat at the feet of Bapuji for hours every day and tried to

quench my spiritual thirst. But Bapuji would tell me again and
again that, 'You will not understand the true value and the full
significance of what you have learned until you reach these levels
yourself." During my stay, Bapuji once mentioned to me, with
overwhelming love, 'It is a grace of God and divine guidance that I
am opening to you the deep and hidden meanings of yoga. In the
past, I have never trained any disciple so intensively, sparing six
hours a day. I enjoy teaching you like I never have in the past'."
(*The Life of Yogi Amrit Desai*, Kripalu Yoga Fellowship, 1982.)

There are two things of significant import happening here.
First, is that their exchange shows how the essence of the guru-disciple relationship is a uniquely unconditional form of human love
that one could make an argument is incomparable to anything else
in the range of adult human relations. (With the exception, of
course, of the first moments parents gaze upon their newborn
baby.) Its rarity and potency makes Amrit Desai, or anyone who
might experience it, long to make it their own, learn how to share it
with others and pass it on. Secondly, and of equal historical
significance, is that Shrii Kripalvanandji is imparting secret or
esoteric knowledge to Amrit Desai, someone whose base of
personal and spiritual activities is not in India.

The latter is significant because before the end of World War II
it was taboo for India to send any of its great sages abroad, or to
export secret teachings to non-Indians, or Indians not making their
home in India. Why? Yogic science has been studying the forces
that make up the imperceptible and invisible world for centuries,
looking for ways to understand and use them toward the amelioration
of the individual and overall human condition. In the last century,

Western science as well has made mind-boggling discoveries about the nature of the 'invisible' world. In both cases, this knowledge can be used toward creative or destructive ends – most notably the use of atoms to completely destroy life as we know it.

It is therefore not a coincidence that the first great Indian sage to come to America, Paramahansa Yogananda (author of *The Autobiography of a Yogi*) did so intentionally at the advent of the nuclear age. From a yogic perspective, the chances of humankind now surviving may very well depend on humanity's ability to alter internal invisible forces creatively in accord with the potency of our newfound capability to use those forces extrinsically and destructively.

Indian sages would no more share their secrets with barbarians than would American nuclear scientists. But now that all the cats have scampered out of their bags (even Schrodinger's), it's just a question of where we will all go with our little and big 'secrets'.

Holy Men, Rich Men & Yogis

Following this intensive period of *sadhana*, Swami Chandra bestowed the title of Yogi upon Amrit Desai. If Amrit Desai was given the title of Yogi just to acknowledge his accomplishments in the study, practice and understanding of yoga then Yogi would be the equivalent of a Masters or Ph.D. in the West.

But the title of Yogi not only recognizes that Amrit Desai has mastered his field of study; it's an *incentive*, an *invitation*, for him to become a Yogi – someone who acquires the attributes, knowledge and powers of a Yogi. Essentially, yogi, like guru, is a state of being, not a title.

The American Nobel Laureate Saul Bellow once wrote a story about a very wealthy and famous man who near the end of his life gave up all his riches to pursue a holy man who was reputed to live simply, serenely, and joyfully. When the rich man finally met up with the holy man the holy man greeted him humbly: 'Great sir, I know what you have sacrificed to come to see me. I only hope that I can say something that will make it worth your effort." The wealthy man looked at him incredulously and replied, "Great sir, I did not come all this way to hear you say *anything*: I came to observe how you tie the laces of your shoes."

Such is the way with Yogis. On one level, they do teach via instruction and intellectual discourse; though on a deeper level they are teaching by embodying the practice and philosophy. It's the years of *sadhana* that has transformed them from ordinary beings into something else. The person is the teaching; not the teaching the person.

The 'Discovery' of Kripalu Yoga

Yogis may perform their yoga *sadhana* by following prescribed blueprints for it, or they may, as Yogi Desai did, forge a new school of yoga based on their personality, place and circumstances.

Yogi Desai is, after all, not living an orthodox yogic lifestyle, surrounded by other yogis and disciples going through various similar stages of *sadhana* in a monastic *ashram*. Yogi Desai is in the throes of an advanced *sadhana*, while at the same time he is married, raising children, running a modern business and living in a proudly secular and pragmatic society. The Yoga he 'discovers' will naturally have to conform equally to his *sadhana*, and his lifestyle.

A brief anecdotal history of yoga will help put Yogi Desai's endeavor into perspective. Most scholars date the beginning of yoga to some 5,000 years ago because archeologists discovered sketches of yoga postures drawn in various places in India at that time. Scholars also tell us that beings in human form with brains about the size of our own have been roaming around the earth for 3 to 4 million years. The root of yoga, or any metaphysics, is to wonder whether or not there is anything more to human life than being born, surviving for a few decades or more, and then expiring and disappearing. I find it hard to believe that human beings – just like us, mentally – went about their business for millions of years without wondering about such things.

Be that as it may, for the sake of putting some time line on this aspect of the story, let's say that yoga as we know it today – with its variety of schools and encyclopedias of instruction – started coming into existence, formally, about five millennia ago. Like most movements connected to its times and culture, it was susceptible to the fluctuations of the society in which it took place. We know that during peaceful and prosperous periods in Indian society it thrived, and that during barbaric ones it was nearly destroyed. That it has managed to survive for thousands of years speaks volumes about its perennial significance and resiliency.

A couple of misconceptions many modern Western practitioners have about yoga, due to the fact that we are receiving it now in a highly structured and homogenized form, is that these schools of Indian yoga must have been concocted over long periods of time, using highly sophisticated applications of research and testing, and then passed on through the ages via scientific and scholarly works. That's true in part, though most schools of yoga originated spontaneously by mystics in primal settings, twisting and contorting extemporaneously in reaction to the metaphysical energies they were entreating, and discovering how to receive, interpret, deal with and incorporate. These individual exhortations and charged movements were observed by others, repeated, investigated, imitated, drawn, copied, made into seals, turned into regimens, passed on, and in time became the specific practiced methodologies and rituals we've come to associate with the different modern schools and disciplines of yoga.

Below the surface of all the formal and external yogic instruction there has always been – in the sects of yoga that have endured, such as the *Pashupats* from which Kripalu is derived – a tradition and practice of internal transformation and external transmission. Internal transformation cannot be adequately described verbally, but it can be shared and discovered through silent observation and active receptiveness. When a yogi or guru transmits spiritual knowledge, it can be felt palpably and taken in viscerally by persons receptive to it.

The 'discovery' of Kripalu Yoga, as you will see, is a perfect example of this esoteric process:

While I was assisting Yogi Desai with the writing of *Kripalu Yoga: Meditation in Motion* (Kripalu Publications, 1985), he recreated his experience of discovering Kripalu Yoga in the following words: "I performed my [yoga] routine with special concentration that morning. A tape-recording of yogic chants by Bapuji played in the background. The intonations of his voice and the gentle accompaniment of the drum stirred feelings of nostalgia and deep reverence within me. As I continued to move, I became absorbed in the rhythm of the chants. Gradually, I became more and more absorbed until I had entered a deep meditative state, even while my body continued to move. My movements had become one with the chanting. Suddenly, as if bursting upon me like an unexpected spring downpour, I was flooded with bliss throughout my entire being, and I felt myself being irresistibly drawn into another level of consciousness. As the music dissolved far into the background, I began feeling that I was no longer the performer of the exercises: they were being performed through me. A new and never-before-experienced flow of energy coursed throughout my system, and with no conscious effort on my part, my body sponta-neously began to twist and turn on its own, flowing smoothly from one posture to the next. The movements were effortless and free, a command and a gift from a newly opened, higher dimension of my inner being. My body became extraordinarily elastic, and stretched smoothly and easily beyond its previous limits. I was not aware of giving any direction to the movements. Thoughts continued to come, but now they passed through my mind in slow motion, seemingly disconnected from my body's activity. Although my eyes were closed, I became distinctly aware that the others in the room had silently stopped their own exercises to watch me. One after another, the postures flowed. Some of them were traditional yoga exercises; others were movements which I had never felt before. At the end of this flow of postures, my body naturally entered the lotus position, and an intense stillness, so deep that it penetrated every level of my being, emanated from within me.

Suddenly, an explosion of ecstasy spread through me, and I became engulfed, overwhelmed, by a state of inner bliss.

About thirty minutes later, my consciousness slowly began to return to normal. With considerable effort, I was able to open my eyes, discovering to my amazement that I was still in my own home surrounded by my wife and friends. It was difficult to move, and my breath was almost imperceptible. My face was completely devoid of expressions, frozen, and immobile. My mouth was dry, and I realized that I had not swallowed for a long time. I tried to speak, but words would not form.

My friends mirrored my trance-like state. As I looked at their unmoving, expressionless eyes, I realized that they, too, had entered a deep state of meditation without closing their eyes. Obviously my experience had communicated itself to them without my saying a word. Gradually and with great difficulty, they began to describe what they had observed while watching me.

Barbara spoke first. Her eyes maintained the unblinking gaze of someone who had just come out of a deep meditation. In a soft, almost inaudible voice, she broke the silence and whispered, 'I felt as if I were doing the postures with you.'

John and my wife nodded in confirmation. They too had experienced it. John spoke haltingly, 'I felt some new energy take you over and move your body. A brilliant light surrounded you. It was a completely new experience for me. I've never seen lights or any such phenomena before.'

Impressed with the consistency of their reactions, I asked Urmilla for her comments. Moved with deep emotion, my wife said, 'It didn't seem as though you were doing the postures. They looked so effortless, as if they were done without your control. They seemed almost -- automatic.'

Automatic? The word rang with a sharp clarity in my mind, evoking the long-forgotten memory of the incident that occurred in India in 1950. I recalled with awe the day Bapuji had taken me into his meditation room. I remembered his remarkable yogic movements: the effortless flowing from one posture to the next with varying degrees of rhythm and tempo."

In that moment, Amrit Desai intuits that his experience parallels that of his guru, an acknowledged master of yoga in India. A spiritual mandate had been issued and received: a new form and practice of yoga is being founded for Americans – not in the ancient rugged foothills of the Himalayas or the modern tony Hollywood Hills, but in a non-descript home in the suburbs of Philadelphia, 1970.

The Beginnings of A New American Yoga? Or What?

Following his experience, Yogi Desai was initially elated, but then became unsure and circumspect about what actually happened. The advanced yogic texts he read informed him that the automatic movements he experienced were a manifestation of a stage in *sadhana* referred to as *samadhi,* in which a practitioner suddenly awakens to increasing amounts of spiritual life force, and is overwhelmed by an initial, primal sense of intimate connection with the cosmos. Yogi Desai associated those kinds of experiences as happening only to yogis who had renounced the world and dedicated themselves exclusively to spiritual practices, as Swami Chandra had done. What did it mean to *his* life? He was a husband, father, teacher, and business person.

Yogi Desai elaborated on his thoughts about his experience as we continued on with *Kripalu Yoga: Meditation in Motion*: "Was my experience similar to what I had witnessed in Bapuji's meditation room? Was it the result of the awakened *pranic* (life force/breath) energy within me? This was hard for me to believe. I had always assumed that a flow of automatic body movements such as this implied an absence of all thought. Yet, I had had thoughts during my experience. Thus, I concluded that my experience could not have been the same automatic performance of exercises. And yet, what was the explanation? Intrigued, and anxious to clarify what had happened to me, I wrote to Bapuji for his interpretation and guidance."

Yogi Desai is experiencing the same dichotomy of thought and feeling that many of his contemporary practitioners of yoga in the West are. How do these metaphysical experiences relate to a 'real' life? Does one need to drop everything they've known previous to explore this new and enticing realm of experience?

Shrii Kripalvanandji wrote back the following:

"My son, your experience was indeed the result of the awakening of your *pranic* energy. This awakening can happen by the grace of God, guru, or through the study and practice of yogic scriptures. As a result of the awakening of *prana*, the body begins to perform postures, breathing exercises, and other *kriyas* (spontaneous movements). These *kriyas* purify the body and mind. During your visit to India last year, I gave you special yogic practices along with specific instruction for their use. Even though these techniques were meant to awaken *prana*, I had withheld their purpose from

you. Due to your appropriate practice of these techniques, you
have been fortunate to receive the benediction of the awakening of
prana, known as *pranotthana*.' (*The States of Kundalini Yoga*,
Shrii Kripalvanandji, Kripalu Yoga *Ashram*, 1975.)

If one is looking for a concrete example of how the esoteric
teachings in yoga work, one has to look no further than the example
of Yogi Desai returning from India initiated as a Yogi and soon
after, 'discovering' a new school of yoga that will transform not only
him, but countless thousands of others.

CHAPTER 5:

GRACE HUSBANDED

The First Kripalu Ashram

I n the winter of 1971, following his *prana* awakening experience, Yogi Desai began cutting back on the number of yoga classes he was teaching, and started spending more time at a rural property he had purchased two years earlier in Sumneytown, Pennsylvania. In his last communiqué, Shrii Kripalvanandji informed Yogi Desai that he had given him full *Shaktipat Diksha* during his last visit because he felt Yogi Desai was now ready to enter *sadhana*.

However, the deeper Yogi Desai went into his practice of yoga, the more his students wanted to be around him. Several even followed him to Sumneytown and moved in with him. In order to be true to his own yoga practice, while at the same time facilitating the sincere desire on the part of his yoga students for a more intensive yoga experience – something he was inspiring in them – he realized that he had to develop a unique approach that combined the two equally.

Yogi Desai: "My highest realization came when I recognized that my path was already unfolding through a slightly different direction than Bapuji's (Shrii Kripalvanandji). My *sadhana* was Kripalu Yoga, flowing with life as it manifested moment to moment. It was neither a complete renunciation nor the usual worldly life. It was a very practical method to bring the mystical experiences of meditation into daily life." (*The Life of Yogi Amrit Desai*, Kripalu Publications, 1982.)

When I asked Yogi Desai what this transitional period was like for him, he told me. "After my experience of going deeper into my yoga practice, I became quieter. I didn't withdraw, but social interactions didn't interest me the same way they had before. And I was also no longer interested in teaching more and more yoga classes. Many people were taking yoga classes because it was something new to try, or because they wanted to lose weight. I mostly wanted to go deeper into my practice. And to surround myself with others who wanted to do the same."

I think it's worthy to note that at this time Yogi Desai could have returned to India as a titled Yogi and premier disciple of Shrii Kripalvanandji, and been given an already established *ashram* in which to pursue his *sadhana*. Though if he did, he would have been bound by traditional Indian cultural restraints, including biases against 'householders' – married persons with families – holding such titled positions and being housed in *ashrams*. (It's not unusual for householders to become yogis and gurus after they fulfill their duties as householders, but rarely at the same time.) In America, Yogi Desai can personally guide his students in Kripalu yoga, enjoy his family, creatively direct the community and, along with them, explore and develop its enterprise. As we've seen so far in this story, it's inimical to Amrit Desai's nature to take the sure or conventional path. A popular adage in the vernacular of this period, the 1970s, is 'do your own thing', and mister Yogi Desai is doing just that.

Yogi Desai Becomes Gurudev:

The early years of The Pennsylvania Yoga Society were for those who enlisted, including many who would remain in the Kripalu community for twenty or more years, the halcyon days of their lives. Yogi Desai, his family, and the young Americans who joined them approached the formidable challenge of creating a viable cross cultural community in the woods of Pennsylvania with great gusto – unbridled optimism, spirited determination, enterprising problem-solving, and heartfelt joy. The property itself stood before them as a great challenge: over 20 acres of hilly, rocky land that had gone to seed. The raw landscape was covered with boulders, brittle thick pines, and thorny scrub brush. The residents would first have to clear it, and then build a dormitory for themselves. The pre-Revolutionary home Yogi Desai and his family lived in, which they shared with his yoga students, had not been lived in for a couple of generations, and would have to be completely restored. And, finally, a large empty stone storage garage without heat or running water needed to be transformed into an attractive central meeting place to host guests.

To accomplish these tasks, residents and Yogi Desai worked side by side, putting in long days together. Yogi Desai taught by

example what he learned by growing up in a small village living
with simple means. (A way of life that none of his middle-class
American counterparts could have even imagined.) As a result, he
approached and led their tasks with a meticulous, frugal and inspiring combination of patience, humility, positive-mindedness, cheer-
fulness and dogged persistence. Together, they turned up floors and
laid carpets, poured cement for walks, rebuilt what they could and
built over what they could not, plastered and painted walls and
ceilings. Additionally, each morning Yogi Desai would lead them
in yoga and meditation practices (*sadhana*), and in the evenings,
communal devotional services that included chanting and dancing
(*satsanga*).

It was around this time that Yoga Society members began to
recognize that Amrit Desai was someone special. They experienced
him not only as a hard working hands-on catalyst for their spiritual
and worldly ambitions, but they also recognized that at the same
time Yogi Desai was becoming one of the most popular and sought
after spiritual teachers of his generation. He had surrendered his
personal ambitions in order to help them create a viable community
for themselves and, in turn, their gratitude gradually began to allow
them to let go of their previous ideas of who they thought they
were, should be, and what their families and society felt they
should do.

As their admiration for Yogi Desai increased, so too did their
attachment. The innate confidence he displayed for his and their
unorthodox mission was something they could only approximate,
so they therefore had to trust in him that together they could make
it work. In time he became for them, organically, no longer just a

teacher, or coworker. But what?

As people more steeped in yogic tradition began flocking to the *ashram* and addressing Yogi Desai as Gurudev, the traditional Sanskrit designation for a guru, so too did the Yoga Society members. Although it at first seems like a simple and affectionate designation, the word 'guru' is so loaded -- with fantasy, misconception, enigma and distortion that Yogi Desai (and his community) will struggle, to this day, about how to relate to it, or not. Adding to the cultural awkwardness of being an Indian guru in America, with American disciples, is that this process was taking place at a time of ultra anti-establishment and anti-authoritarian sentiment in American society. Furthermore, most Pennsylvania Yoga Society members – unlike their counterparts in India – were not coming to Sumneytown in order to 'find their guru', or become part of an Indian yogic lineage, or even embark on a serious spiritual practice. The name Gurudev for most of these original American 'disciples' was a term of affection and endearment rather than the designation of a serious commitment that the word carried in Indian culture.

Michael Richards, one of the first Sumneytown residents, described his experience this way: "I first saw Gurudev (Amrit Desai) when I walked into his yoga class at the First Unitarian Church in Philadelphia in 1970. I suddenly felt a special bond. When he purchased the property in Sumneytown, I thought of moving in, but was drawn to living half of my life with friends, work, and autonomy in Philadelphia, and half in pursuit of self-realization in the contemplative environment of the *ashram*. I questioned whether this growing relationship with Amrit would, like other relationships, eventually prove to be less than what I really wanted in life. However, as Amrit's teaching about Swami Kripalvananda and yoga intensified, the pull I felt to the *ashram* grew. Observing his equanimity during and following interactions that would normally be emotionally upsetting to most of us, I had come to trust Amrit, and eventually I moved in." (In an email from Michael Richards, 6/8/09.)

Michael Richards, an architectural designer, would become an administrator in the first Kripalu Ashram. More than thirty years later, he is still personally and professionally affiliated with The Kripalu Center in Massachusetts.

Yogi Desai Rediscovers de Toqueville's America:

In the charmed early years of the Pennsylvania Yoga Society, Yogi Desai was recreating Alexis de Toqueville's America for himself and his cohorts. Rather than using the Indian model for forming *ashrams* around a yogi or guru in a culture that broadly promoted and supported such things, the Pennsylvania Yoga Society was following the classic and distinctly American blueprint for creating new enterprise: an energetic and ambitious immigrant as the catalyst, an enthusiastic young American workforce, and a network of open-minded civic groups supporting their activities. A look back at Yogi Desai's itinerary from this time finds him driving around the greater Philadelphia area in a yellow '65 Chevy Impala offering lectures on Indian philosophy, and providing demonstrations of Kripalu Yoga at Unitarian churches, Elks and Rotary Clubs, YMCAs, community colleges, school gymnasiums, and virtually any venue that would have him.

Yogi Desai was living The American Dream in a way few

Americans were still doing then, and hardly do any longer. If Kripalu Yoga was discovered by someone with Yogi Desai's credentials today, more likely a group of investors would create a virtual *ashram* for him, launch an interactive website, and then bring in revenues by offering online classes and seminars. Not work it up personally from Main Street the way Yogi Desai and his family and students are doing.

When the Desai family permanently moved onto the property in Sumneytown in the winter of 1972, Yogi Desai formally designated his home as an *ashram* and invited five of his yoga students, all male, to join him and live there full-time. When female students objected to this quarantine as being 'discriminatory' – this was, after all, 20th century America, not ancient India – he also agreed to allow five women to move in. Thus began the first co-ed residential Kripalu Ashram in America.

As one would expect, Yogi Desai and his followers will experience some major Big MACS: Mutually Assured Culture Shocks.

America in the 1970's

The 1970s, if you recall, were a time of monumental social and political turmoil and change in America. The war in Vietnam finally concluded as strangely as it began, but not before taking the lives of scores of Vietnamese, tens of thousands of young Americans, and bringing on the most critical social and political imbroglio in America since the Civil War. Black Americans burned down cities from Newark to Watts in 1967 and '68, and the nation felt to many as though it was on an inevitable fast-track to either an apartheid society or a full scale race war. The birth-control pill liberated women from the tyranny of the fear of sex and pregnancy, and in the process helped turn over more than two thousand years of repressive Judeo-Christian constructs regarding sexual behavior and gender roles. It was within this atmosphere that young 60's wayfarers began finding their way into the orbit of Yogi Amrit Desai. (Two of the original members of the Sumneytown *Ashram* told me that they'd "just stopped in to check out this guru thing" before heading on to either Haight-Ashbury or Greenwich Village.)

This is my generation I am talking about, so I feel confident in speaking generally, though personally, about what we were doing at that time and how we felt about it. We had no idea that the lifestyle choices we were making, and the political and social activism we were engaged in, was going to create the kinds of havoc on, and misunderstandings from, American society that it did. Our outlook was defined more by what we were against than what we were for. We were against the Vietnam War, against sexual repression and gender discrimination, and against racism. But most of us had no idea what we were for, or how to get there. (The assassinations of many of our political and civil rights leaders in the 1960's did not help secure direction.) This obstinate and confrontational stance against the mainstream of society, or what we referred to then as 'The Establishment', coupled with a lack of direction about what else to do, or who else to ally ourselves with, bred intense feelings of alienation, insecurity and confusion. We were looking for new ways of thinking and acting, and experimenting in our lifestyles in ways that felt natural. Most of us could not share our thoughts and feelings with Depression-era parents who were dreadfully frightened and threatened by any movement on our part away from the economic security of the status-quo.

Our generation inspired the phrase 'generation gap', and our parents and we deserved it. In the 1970's, young Americans felt like refugees from their own culture, their own families. We were desperately looking for safe places in which to explore self-expression and feel empathy. Eastern mysticism and spiritual communities were among the attractive alternatives.

Indian spiritualism was particularly attractive to many of us because, it was, unlike our own Judeo-Christian heritage that was built upon ten commandments for living a short, clean life in arduous times, born during one of the most creative and prosperous periods in Indian history. Therefore, it offered a deluxe outlook on life that was wondrous, open, dynamic, playful, and refreshingly optimistic. Its philosophy celebrated life in the here and now, with a unique cosmic construct that described the creation of the universe not as being the result of a benignly authoritarian God rubbing pieces of clay together, nor by a 'Big Bang' of previously inert and 'non-existing' elements somehow coming together accidentally; but by the willful and joyful union of Shiva and Shakti, the male and female principles of Divinity. The 'Big Bang' was not a mechanical accident; it was a 'Grand Orgasm'. Life was created lovingly, sexually, wildly and ecstatically. Now imagine yourself in your twenties, enjoying your first sexual experiences, smoking a little pot, and hearing that?!

It wasn't gurus, or alternative authority figures we were chasing, it was an outlook toward life that included wonder, harmony, excitement and joy.

Disciple Means Discipline?

Amrit Desai, as we've noted, was born for the role he was moving into as an adult. He was self-directed, purposeful, and he also had the extraordinary good fortune at an early age of meeting one of India's most accomplished yoga adepts who personally guided him though an intensive spiritual practice as a young man. Afterward, Amrit Desai dutifully accepted an arranged marriage, and with it, the responsibilities of being a husband and father. His background was, simply put, the antithesis of what most young Americans were living at this time, or wanted to be living.

An anecdote told to me by Yogi Desai's son Malay illustrates the initial interface between Yogi Desai and his young American disciples. Malay was eight or nine years old when the Sumneytown *ashram* started up in the early 70s. It was his custom to awaken with his dad early in the morning and go with him from the basement, where his family was sleeping in their own home, to the first floor, where *ashram* residents were staying. Yogi Desai would try to engage them in some kind of morning activity as a precursor to yoga practice – just a short jog or brisk walk. *Anything.* On one such occasion, Malay Desai recalled, with a smile, "My dad wasn't having much luck. His appeals were met with moans and groans that sounded mostly like "no". Except for one guy with long hair who was staring down at a guitar on his lap. He looked up at my dad and said, 'Sure, man, as soon as I finish tuning up.'"

Yogi Desai recalled those times this way: "The early 70s were the height of 'new age' values; lots of hugging, being mellow and not taking responsibility. People were not looking for in-depth spiritual disciplines like a person who was entering a monastery. Many were trying to escape from life's challenges. Others were looking for a natural high." (*The Life of Yogi Amrit Desai,* Kripalu Publications, 1982.)

So from Yogi Desai's perspective, Kripalu Yoga was the perfect vehicle for his in-home resident/disciples to become grounded in the spiritual lifestyle they professed to be seeking – by practicing it. Kripalu Yoga and the *ashram* lifestyle would provide them with a comprehensive and methodical approach to developing physically, mentally and emotionally. The practice of the yoga postures would provide them with strength and discipline, meditation would help clear and focus their minds, and communal living would engage them socially. Additionally, Yogi Desai was able to offer *shaktipat* as a way to gracefully aid their adjustment from spiritual adolescence to maturity.

The latter stratagem, however, was not having the effect Yogi Desai anticipated, or wanted. "At first, this (giving *shaktipat*) seemed to be the answer to my intense desire to share my blissful experience with others. For a while I closely observed all those who experienced *prana* awakening through contact with me, and who had many ecstatic meditative experiences of spontaneous postures and other involuntary movements. However, those people consistently exposed to *prana shakti* also experienced so much intense emotional catharsis and physical purification that it affected their ability to carry out their normal daily responsibilities. They were often moody and irritable, and also found that their sexual energy became overactive." (*Kripalu Yoga: Meditation-In-Motion* Kripalu Publications, 1985.)

Yogi Desai later added this observation (same source): "I eventually stopped the outward flow of *shakti* energy because so many were not ready to handle the intensity of the physical, mental and emotional purification that it brings. I realized that my disciples needed more grounding, more clarity in their thoughts and emotions, and more purification in their bodies before moving to this deeper level. Bapuji was realizing similar things in his work in India, and he wrote to me: 'Do not give *shaktipat* except to a few disciples.' I had come to the same conclusion."

So Yogi Desai returned to his basic blueprint: that the consistent practice of yoga and meditation combined with a simple and responsible lifestyle was required in order for his disciples to move along further with their personal and spiritual development. This also followed more accurately his own experience; he'd practiced yoga and meditation for more than twenty years before he had a spiritual awakening experience that he was mature enough to understand and make useful purpose of. And it was only afterward that he received *shaktipat* from his guru in order to strengthen his already apparent resolve, and in the process open him to deeper spiritual understanding and experiences.

Even in fast-paced America, it turned out, there could be no shortcuts. Therefore, the first thing Yogi Desai wanted to teach his young disciples was how to be disciplined, or how to practice. (The word disciple derives from discipline.) And specifically, what he wanted them to learn, and make the foundation of their lives, was the practice of Kripalu Yoga.

As with any true form of yoga or spiritual practice, the aim of Kripalu Yoga is to develop skills and attributes that extend well

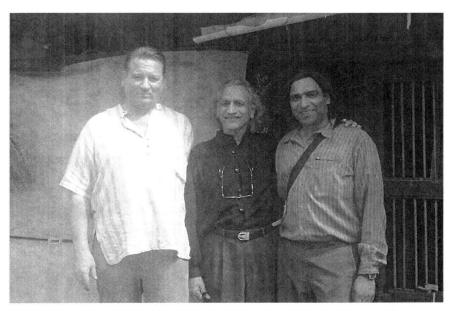

Author James Abro with Yogi Amrit Desai, the Founder of Kripalu Yoga and his son, Malay. Picture taken in the Indian village where Yogi Desai grew up.

beyond the purpose of the exercise or practice. The overall purpose of practicing Kripalu Yoga is to incorporate the benefits of increased strength, endurance, flexibility, and mental focus into an ethical, creative, inner directed and self-disciplined way of life. As Yogi Desai was fond of telling his students, "Don't focus on making money, or getting into relationships, and all of that. Just focus on your spiritual practices and the rest will come easily and naturally." (*Working Miracles of Love*, Kripalu Publications, 1990.)

But how do yoga students learn to become more self-assured, creative, and independent-minded by applying practices given to them by someone else? Yogi Desai related how the continued practice of yoga itself allowed him to move from a mechanical practice and understanding of yoga, and life, into an approach that was more open, creative, spontaneous and dynamic. "In spite of all the knowledge of yoga I had acquired over a long period of study, I had never been able to tune into my own needs with such precision (as after I had my *prana*-awakening experience). Previously, I had practiced a fixed routine, a traditional approach to yoga postures and hardly paid any attention to my body's needs. I discovered that this intelligence of *prana* knew what to do, how long to hold a posture, and what the next movement would be. All choices and movements of postures originated from somewhere deep within my body and were precisely designed to meet my needs on any given day at any given time. There was no set sequence. Each day my body's internal needs chose new combinations and postures. The familiar routine and traditional way of practice became secondary, and the inner wisdom of the body that came in the form of urges that guided and choreographed the movements became primary. This made my daily practice a refreshing experience, a new and constant source of joy for me." (*Kripalu Yoga: Meditation in Motion*. Kripalu Publications, 1985.)

Contemporary chemical biologists are discovering that amino acids 'fold' into proteins in order to create the vast and various cells that make up our bodies. This mysterious 'folding' process takes place within the body in a matter of tiny fractions of a second -- to decide, adapt and execute whether to become a bone cell or, say, a liver cell. Scientists attempting to duplicate a single folding-selection process using supercomputers found that it would take them 10 to the 27th power number of years to duplicate one process, given all the options. That's a billion times a billion times a billion years. ("Proteins 1, Computers 0," *The New York Times*, 12/19/03.)

The experience of an 'inner wisdom of the body' Yogi Desai made in the process of discovering Kripalu Yoga is significant for two specific reasons. One, it elevates the practice of Kripalu Yoga beyond the purely mechanical physical practice of postures; and two, by recognizing that the postures are not the be all and end all, it makes Kripalu Yoga complementary with many other practices and techniques -- ancient and modern -- designed not only for maintaining health and well-being, but for enhancing intuition, creativity and knowledge.

But Kripalu Yoga, like any other discipline, requires commitment and consistent practice before any tangible, let alone extraordinary, gains can be realized.

Jazz & Yoga

Kripalu Yoga, an American spiritual practice with roots in another culture, Indian, lends itself well to comparison with Jazz, an American art form with roots in Africa. Fully developed, both require a sound understanding and virtuoso accomplishment of the basics of their discipline, and along with that, the willingness, courage and intelligence to depart from the form and improvise on one's own.

As Yogi Desai, and other teachers have learned, it's not easy to teach people to improvise, to think on their feet. The primary stumbling block being that most people are schooled to learn by rote or through imitation, reinforced by a stark fear of doing things incorrectly or inadequately. Within this punitive educational gestalt, spontaneity and originality are often so rare that, as we shall see, even when observed, experienced and encouraged, they are only mimicked.

The first piece of the puzzle that Yogi Desai felt he had to put together was to find a method to teach a sophisticated, intuitive, and spontaneous form of yoga to students who were just beginning to learn the fundamentals of doing yoga postures. Yogi Desai concluded that he needed a way to *show* his students what he meant by Kripalu Yoga, rather than just tell them. He came up with what he called a 'posture flow'. A posture flow is done by first entering into a quiet and still state of meditation, and then allowing *prana*, or one's life force, to direct the flow of movements that follow. The purpose of this exercise is to circumvent the usually over-riding dictates of the mind, and thus allow the practitioner to find other sources of knowledge and wisdom within themselves. (Modern neurobiologists recently discovered that there is as much, or more, neurological activity taking place in the heart, and other organs of the body, as the brain, refuting the long-held assumption that the brain is the sole, largest and most important command center in the human body. (*The Biology of Transcendence*, Joseph Chilton Pearce, Park Street Press, 2003.)

The benefits of practicing yoga in this inner-directed fashion include being much less likely to strain or hurt oneself by getting into a willful competition with one's own, or other peoples' minds and bodies. And you are also more likely to emerge from the experience feeling an increase in self-confidence and trust.

The posture flow is also pleasant to watch and do. Watching the posture flow performed by Yogi Desai, or any advanced Kripalu Yoga practitioner, is like listening to Duke Ellington or Miles Davis improvise over a standard.

After Yogi Desai developed this method for demonstrating Kripalu Yoga and executed it in front of his students, he was surprised, though not discouraged, to find students duplicating his posture flow -- exactly, move for move.

The irascible jazz bassist Charlie Mingus described this phenomena when he titled one of his compositions as an homage to the memory of Charlie Parker, the prodigiously improvisational saxophonist who was copied note for note by a whole generation of musicians: "If Charlie Parker Was a Gunslinger\ There'd Be a Lot of Dead Imitators."

The Kripalu Ashram becomes an Artist Colony for Aspiring Yogis

Undeterred, Yogi Desai realized, once again, as with offering *shaktipat*, that there would be no shortcuts in the process of training students to practice yoga, not only as a practical way of improving the quality of their lives, but also as a spontaneous and personal path toward spiritual fulfillment.

He realized that he'd have to create a place where he and his students could feel free to explore this new form of yoga, and with it, new found qualities and attributes within themselves. In effect, by founding the Kripalu Yoga *Ashram* dedicated to establishing a new improvisational form of yoga, Yogi Desai was establishing the first American artist colony for aspiring yogis.

But what about S-E-X?

By far, the most contentious and problematic issue Yogi Desai had to face in establishing this unorthodox co-ed Indian-style *ashram* in the sylvan woods of Pennsylvania, is what kind of lifestyle to recommend. The only model for *ashram* life Yogi Desai was familiar with was the one practiced in India: the residents do spiritual practices in the morning and evening; during the day work voluntarily as a form of *seva* or selfless service and eat a nutritious though meatless diet. Non-married men and women, regardless of their personal sexual propensities, were to live apart and not engage in sexual relations. This is the model he proposed, and to which the residents tried to adapt.

Other alternative spiritual communities starting up at this time, most notably the Dawn Horse Communion and The Farm (both founded, not coincidentally, by Americans) were not demanding such conservative lifestyles, especially in regard to sexual activity. Being Americans, Gaskin (The Farm) and Da Free John (Dawn Horse) more easily recognized the positive and irrepressible aspects of the 'sexual revolution' that was taking place in American society at this time, and encouraged openness, intimacy and experimentation in their communities. Amrit Desai, on the other hand, had been in the United States only a little more than a decade, and grew up in a part of the world where arranged marriages and sexual fidelity were still the lynchpins for social and economic stability. He simply did not have any personal or social reference to aid him in understanding the significance and importance of the sexual liberation politics of this time, and how it related to the larger issues of gender

equality and personal freedom so important to this generation of
Americans.

The choice of lifestyle created a simmering hotbed of tension
and unexpressed conflict between Amrit Desai and the Kripalu
community that would be ongoing and last through all the predictable
phases of repression and excess, until it ended up becoming both
an integral part of the exceptional growth of the Kripalu enterprise,
as well as its near downfall. As a result of residents sublimating
their sexual drive in favor of yoga and work, it made the community
extraordinarily productive. Though, at the same time, it also created
an acceptable form of escape from personal intimacy, interrupting the
personal development of many young residents, as well as making
others deny their feelings or hide their activities.

I think it is important to note that Yogi Desai did not propose
these lifestyle guidelines to his students in order to repress them, or
to gain authority over them. To the best of his knowledge and experience, at the time, the lifestyle he was advocating for the residents of the *ashram* was the most effective way he knew of for
them to get the most out of the spiritual practices he was offering.

Many residents over the years accepted the lifestyle guidelines
temporarily in order to get the most out of an immersion in a yogic
spiritual lifestyle. They then went on to incorporate those benefits
into the life they were living previously. Others accepted and
enrolled in the *ashram's* 'marriage program', whereby after four
years of residency one could go through a supervised period of
courtship with a resident of equal tenure, and, if it worked out,
marry. The lifestyle guidelines became problematic for the residents who tried to make them their permanent lifestyle – thinking

that they were in synch with Yogi Desai, who openly advocated the spiritual benefits of celibacy.

The conflict this causes later when residents learn that Yogi Desai has been less than honest with them about his own sexual behavior will nearly bring down the Kripalu enterprise and Yogi Desai; though, fortunately, both the Kripalu community and Yogi Desai managed to get through it and move on successfully in their own ways.

As we shall see, it's one thing to discover a new brand of yoga; and it's quite another to maintain a practice of it through life's vicissitudes. To their credit, both Yogi Desai and the core members of the Kripalu community do just that.

The Kripalu Yoga Fellowship

As Yogi Desai's reputation as a vibrant new spiritual teacher began to grow, so too did the demand for his seminars, appearances and demonstrations of Kripalu Yoga. People were literally dropping in from all over the world to check out this new guru. These are Yogi Desai's thoughts about that time: "Up until 1974, I personally owned the *ashram* and everything in it. I saw that my personal profit was going to increase dramatically as large numbers of people came here to attend programs. I didn't want to be a businessman and involve my energies in moneymaking. I told Michael Risen and Sandra Healy (two of the original resident\disciples; Risen a lawyer; Healy a businesswoman) to turn the whole organization into a non-profit trust that would benefit the work. Then I handed over the entire organization to the Kripalu Yoga Fellowship. I relinquished all personal profit, and simply took a yearly salary to support my family and myself."

Despite the apparently benign intentions, the Kripalu Yoga Fellowship was, in effect, set up to support a hierarchy of one: it named Yogi Desai its spiritual director, and also made him its sole salaried employee. Residents of the *ashram* would not be paid salaries until Kripalu was restructured after Yogi Desai's departure in 1994. Up until then, despite the extraordinary financial success of The Kripalu Center for Yoga and Health, the staff\residents, in accordance with traditional *ashram* policy, were paid modest monthly living stipends, plus room and board.

An unforeseen byproduct of Yogi Desai's arrangement with The Kripalu Yoga Fellowship was that The Fellowship now owned all the physical and intellectual properties belonging to Kripalu, including Kripalu Yoga.

But in 1974, there were only clear skies and sunshine on the foreseeable horizon. No one then could have been able to predict either the phenomenal successes that the Kripalu Center and Yogi Desai would achieve, nor the bitter split that would take place between them. At this point in the story, Yogi Desai and his disciples are too busy gingerly husbanding Grace.

CHAPTER 6:

GRACE BREAKS TOO HARD AND MISCUES

Shakti Guru

A Yogi receiving *shaktipat diksha*, and the ability to transmit *shaktipat*, is afterward highly regarded and sought out.

A Yogi with these capacities is known as a Shakti Guru. The Shakti Guru is not marked by this new-found attribute in any noticeable external way. They may feel six inches taller, their eyes may brighten, complexions glow sanguine, and they may exude a warmth or heat -- but these manifestations are too similar to what occurs from a good day at the spa to be note-worthy to a casual observer. The changes that do take place are internal and sublime, and are generally picked up only by people who, for whatever reasons, are drawn to it. And these people often have dramatic reactions.

Yogi Desai experienced this kind of response for the first time publicly when he was invited to speak at the annual Spiritual Frontiers

Fellowship in Chicago, shortly after returning to America from India. The following are some of the observations and reactions he recorded right after that appearance: "At the Spiritual Frontiers Fellowship lecture, I didn't understand how what I said could have commanded such a response from the audience. People were in tears, and many looked as though they had been stunned. A great number told me that they had seen lights around me. I was amazed at their response." (*The Life of Yoga Amrit Desai*, Kripalu Yoga Fellowship, 1985.)

Within the American counter-culture at this time there was a vital subculture focused not so much on young longhaired British rockers mimicking American soul and blues music, as they were on the metaphysical and spiritual exploits of some of the literary notables and social icons of the time. This group memorized Allen Ginsburg's *Howl*, aspired to be members of Jack Keroac's *Dharma Bums* and observed John Lennon (the peacenik, not the 'Beatle') returning from India transcendentally 'turned on' in 1969. They also listened raptly to John Coltrane's *Love Supreme* and adhered to Timothy Leary's post-modern proclamation to 'turn on and drop out.'

This subculture traveled a circuit that included visits to Swami Shrii Rudrananda in New York City; to California to see Long Island born Bubba Free John; they spent time at The Farm with Stephen Gaskin in Tennessee (where smoking marijuana was a requirement for residency); as well as stopovers with Philip Kapleau at the Zen Center in Rochester, New York; Swami Shrii Kriyananda at the Ananda *Ashram*, California; Baker Roshi at Tassajara Zen Center in Big Sur; Swami Shrii Muktananda at his upstate New York *Ashram*; and now, Yogi Amrit Desai in Sumneytown, Pennsylvania.

One of the ways the public gauged the potency and authenticity of their prospective gurus was in the ability of these gurus to deliver *shaktipat*. *Shaktipat* can feel like a mild electrical charge going through the body, or like the first stages of a drug or alcohol induced high, or sexual anticipation: it arouses the senses. Receiving a dose of it is usually accompanied by feelings of stimulation, serenity and, sometimes, euphoria. Those who are receptive to it generally have experienced something like it previously in their lives, by ways that I just mentioned, or other means – but rarely by simply sitting in the presence of someone.

If you are open to it, *shaktipat* is the cotton candy you can get right at the opening to an exotic cosmic fairground of practices and rituals designed to return you to a heightened and more enjoyable experience of *Life*. As Jesus Christ (no doubt a Shakti Guru) put it: I came that they may have life, and have It abundantly." [John 10:10] *Shaktipat* is the energetic key that opens the body and mind to an abundant reservoir of higher mental, physical and psychic powers, releasing blissful emotional feelings along the way.

Yogi Desai was offering *shaktipat* because he thought that transmitting it would allow his students to integrate it into their practice and lives as he had done. And at the same time allow him to spend more time with his spiritual practices or *sadhana*. The personal dilemma for Yogi Desai at this time is how to manage the power of this spiritual force, in others and in himself. One can readily imagine that the charged energy of *shaktipat* that others are feeling so strongly from Yogi Desai is also happening within him to an even greater degree.

Unlike Shrii Kripalvanandji, who practiced a private and

secluded *sadhana* for many decades before he was made spiritual director of an *ashram* with disciples in India, Yogi Desai is being thrust into the role of spiritual teacher and Shakti Guru at the same time he is raising a family, directing a business, and adapting to a new and unfamiliar culture. In the span of one decade, Amrit Desai moved to another country, fathered three children, graduated college, pursued a brief though successful art career, discovered a new school of yoga, founded a Yoga Society and was initiated in India as a Yogi. As an adult, in America, it has been difficult for Amrit Desai to find private time for himself, let alone his *sadhana*.

A Pivotal Year:

1974 started out quietly, with Yogi Amrit Desai finally getting the opportunity he had been longing for since returning from India; to be able to practice yoga *sadhana* in seclusion for a while.

The Kripalu Ashram now had more than forty residents and a waiting list for that many more. Together, the original forty residents first built a dormitory facility for themselves and then shortly afterward began constructing a separate, self-contained structure secluded in a wooded area for the purpose of accommodating Yogi Desai for a three-month period of seclusion and *sadhana*. They named the airy, two-story building *Muktidham*, the Abode of Liberation.

Yogi Desai's period of seclusion had two primary benefits. One, it allowed the residents and staff an opportunity to manage the *ashram* and themselves without his supervision. The residents learned that it was one thing to live a 'spiritual lifestyle' when you are being told to do so by an authority figure, and quite another to maintain that lifestyle on your own without outside pressure and guidance. Several residents found that being left on their own was not the way they wanted to live, and took their leave in his absence, though the majority of residents made it their choice to stay. These steadfast residents would become the mainstays of the Kripalu community and enterprise for the next few decades, as well as become the executives who would administer its highly successful operations.

Yogi Desai, characteristically, derived simple and practical benefit from the experience: "From my childhood I had a fear of being alone in the dark, where there were no people around to help me in case I was in trouble. (When Amrit Desai was nine-years-old he experienced a nearly fatal bout of typhoid.) Until I went into Muktidham, I carried this fear, but was never in a situation to allow it to surface and be worked out. Suddenly, there I was, all alone in the woods, and this same fear came up during my first night. I became very focused on it and said to myself, 'In all these years, how often have I felt this fear, and known that it never became a reality?' Instantly, with this realization, I decided not to think these fearful thoughts, and it never once came up for me again. I dropped it right then and there and went to sleep. God gave me life. He can take it in the way He wants to take it." (*Gurudev: The Life of Yogi Amrit Desai*, Kripalu Publications, 1982.)

How Sarasvati Chandra Became a Swami:

In 1974, Yogi Desai would also receive another invitation from Shrii Kripalvanandji, this time to attend the commemoration of the completed restoration of the Temple in Kayavarohan. In Chapter 3,

I noted that the Temple of Kayavarohan had been razed by
Moslem invaders in the 11th century CE and that Swami Chandra
had been told by his guru that he would restore it. I described
then how it basically came about, but seeing that it is such a fantastic
story, and pertinent to the background of the emergence of Kripalu
Yoga, I will provide more details now.

As a young man, Shrii Kripalvanandji (nee Sarasvati Chandra)
was possessed by a single-minded passion to achieve intimate
union with God. By the tender age of nineteen, Chandra had
become so frustrated by his inability to achieve this goal that he
considered suicide.

When Sarasvati Chandra was on his way to attempt this dire
act, a man he'd never seen or met before stopped him. To Chandra's
amazement, the stranger knew his darkest thoughts and intentions.
The nameless stranger then ordered Chandra to follow him to an
ashram. The *ashram* Chandra was escorted to was one of the finest
in Bombay, catering to its wealthy and social elite. To Chandra's
further amazement, the congregation at the *ashram* welcomed him
as though they'd been expecting him. Four months earlier, it had
been 'forecast' that on this day a young man would appear at this
ashram who would become one of India's most accomplished
yogis and saints. 'Forecasts' in India are not like Western 'forecasts'
of what weather or economic conditions might be like. In India,
'forecasts' describe conditions *as they are* – whether phenomenal
reality coincides at the moment or not.

Embarrassed by the attention and proclamation, especially in
light of the disreputable way he had been planning on spending
this day, the young man nevertheless humbly agreed to stay and do

whatever the stranger who saved him asked of him.

Chandra, starting the very next day, embarked on an assigned regimen of *sadhana* that must have *seemed* at times like death to the nineteen-year-old. Chandra was secluded from the outside world for a period of a year-and-a-half, during which time he fasted silently for intermittent periods of forty days while being introduced to the rudiments of yogic spiritual practices: meditation, *mantra* (chanting), *asana*, (yoga postures), prayer, reading scriptures and *pranayama* (breathing exercises). More importantly, he received *shaktipat-diksha* from his mentor, the arcane and integral part of the initiation of aspirants into the deepest and most esoteric aspects of yoga.

Following his intensive *sadhana* and *diksha* (initiation), Chandra begged his mentor to tell him more about himself and why he had chosen him. But the mysterious stranger remained steadfastly just that: he would tell Chandra only that "in time you will discover these things for yourself'. They then traveled together to sacred sites in India where they worshipped and prayed. One day, Chandra's guru informed him that within a decade he would renounce the world and take on the saffron robes of a *sannyasin*, or swami.

Chandra vehemently objected to this 'forecast' for a couple of strongly felt reasons. One, Chandra had been born and raised a Brahmin. It deeply offended his vanity and pride to think of himself as ever being a penniless beggar dependent on strangers for sustenance. Secondly, Chandra was educated and had a strong intellect. He'd dismissed these ancient traditions and practices as antiquated, foolish, and devoid of meaning.

The enigmatic stranger then mysteriously disappeared, leaving

Chandra with the promise that they would meet again after Chandra
became a swami. Chandra returned to Bombay where for six years
he pursued a career in music, acting, and playwriting, and also
became engaged to be married. Although he did not attain commercial
success, or marry, the time was not misspent. In the years to follow,
Chandra would write allegorical stories and scholarly texts on yoga
that are considered classics, compose devotional music prodigiously,
and become a popular and eloquent orator on earthy as well as
spiritual matters – including the misappropriations of human love.

After six years of worldly pursuits, Sarasvati Chandra found
himself becoming intensely restless. He was not able to get the
mysterious stranger out of his thoughts or come to terms with why
the man had selected him for yogic training and then just disappeared.
Feeling lummoxed, Chandra embarked on a solitary spiritual
pilgrimage to Rishikesh, a renowned holy site in the lowland
forests and foothills of the Himalayas. While he was walking
toward his destination he passed a man who called out to him in a
moniker only his mysterious mentor had ever used. Chandra's
teacher was about sixty years old the last time he saw him, and this
man appeared vibrant, fit and youthful.

When Chandra looked back at him, the man asked: "Don't you
recognize me?"

In that moment, Chandra recognized that it was his teacher
appearing before him in a perfect, ethereal yogic body. Chandra
supplicated himself at the yogi's feet and begged him to finally
reveal who he was.

The yogi assured Chandra once again that someday soon he
would find that out on his own. He then disappeared once again.

Shortly afterward, Chandra surrendered to the mysterious directives
and took formal vows as a renunciate monk in order to become a
swami.

After taking the vows, Swami Chandra immersed himself in the
sacred texts of Indian literature and once again took up his dedication
to the practice of *sadhana* that had empirically saved his life.
When he felt himself filled with knowledge, and strong enough to
trust that 'God will provide', he embarked on a peripatetic mission
to bring the sacred teachings of India to as many small towns and
villages as his feet could carry him. Being a traveling mendicant
depending on the world to take care of him was, in the beginning,
as difficult for Chandra. In the long run, it would be so beneficial
to his developing such a profound faith in God that he would in
fact elevate his life out of the worldly and ordinary to such a
degree that he would be recognized as a rare master of *Kundalini*
Yoga (the yoga of complete surrender to God).

It was also at about this time, in the late 1940's, when Swami
Chandra wandered into a town called Halol and made such a
remarkable and lasting impression on a shy teenage boy named
Amrit Desai.

Shiva Ratri: Holy Flying Phalluses

Swami Chandra maintained his peripatetic mission, along with
his *sadhana*, for another few years, until the pull of his *sadhana*,
along with the sublime awakening of life force that came as a result
of the *diksha* he received, became so great that it forced him to
retreat into the confines of an *ashram* in order to assimilate what
was happening. He stayed there for a couple of years, practicing a

sadhana that included six hours a day of silence, yoga, meditation and prayer.

He emerged from his self-imposed quarantine a stronger yogi, though there were two questions that remained burning inside of him. What was the identity of his guru, and what temple did his guru want him to restore?

Then, in 1955, as I noted briefly in a section of Chapter 3 called 'The Roots of Kripalu Yoga', Swami Chandra was invited to speak in the village of Kayavarohan during a holy week. The Temple in Kayavarohan is mentioned in the *Puranas*, which date back some 3500 years, as a Maha Shiva Tirtha, or major sacred place for the worship of Lord Shiva.

Earlier I mentioned that the bodily form of Swami Chandra's guru, Lord Lakulish, had merged into a black stone obelisk. That black stone obelisk was one of thirteen large jet-colored shards of meteorites that landed in the vicinity of Kayavarohan 2500 years earlier. (Roughly the same time that Buddha- and Christ-consciousness emerged.) These phallic shaped objects were called *Jyotirlingams* (phalluses of light), considered sacred, and were distributed and displayed prominently in major temples dedicated to the worship of Lord Shiva.

[There is currently a group of scientists calling themselves biochemical evolutionists who are looking for evidence of proof that human consciousness (after all no one has yet proven how we got from chimp brain to here) was tweaked by molecules of living organisms found in objects brought to earth from outer space.] BBC World Report, May 2009.

When Shaivism (or the worshipping of Shiva) began waning in

India in the second century CE, Lord Shiva incarnated as a baby
into a devout Hindu family in the town of Kayavarohan. There, he
literally began leading religious ceremonies from the cradle, died
suddenly, was resurrected from a large body of water. He was then
recognized by local holy men as Lord Lakulish, the twenty-eighth
incarnation of Lord Shiva, or earthly Son of God. Lord Lakulish,
an actual historic figure, founded the Pashupats sect of Shaivism,
which became a major influence on Indian society and culture for
the next 1500 years. Included among its accomplishments was
establishing the Brahmin, or priestly and educated class, and
formalizing the scientific study and practice of yoga. For the latter
accomplishment, Lord Lakulish is regarded as the 'father of yoga'.

During this period, temples to Shiva were erected in almost
every village, while at the same time India became a prosperous
trading center. Grateful royals embossed the image of Lord Lakulish
onto the national coinage. Prior to the invasions of the Moslems
and the imposition of colonialism by the British, it was common in
Indian villages to find stone symbols of lingams (phalluses) and
yonis (vaginas) displayed openly. It was believed that offering
reverential worship to the reproductive process and its organs
brought, among other things, fertility, security, prosperity, serenity
and harmony.

When Lord Lakulish felt that his mission on earth was accomplished – to restore Shaivism – he gathered his disciples together
around the *Jyotirlingam* set on the main altar in the Temple of
Kayavarohan and then asked them to shut their eyes and meditate.
When they opened their eyes, the disciples were astonished to find
that Lord Lakulish had miraculously merged into the *Jyotirlingam*.

I visited the Temple of Kayavarohan in 2007, and it was easy to see why the Moslems would try to destroy it and the British oppress it. The stone façade of its baroque steeples and spires have the forms of females intricately sculpted into them — archetypal depictions of water carriers, gopis, maidens, consorts, attendants. They are either partially dressed or nude, striking enticing poses. There is nothing untoward in the poses or the expressions on the women's faces. They are simply part and parcel of a body of some of the finest, most evocative erotic art ever produced by humans, and it dates back three thousand years.

But what must have been the coup de grace for the Moslem conquistadors, British imperialists, and any unprepared (or prepared) non-Shaivite visitor, is what is on the main altar of the Temple of Kayavarohan. Not only *is* there a life-size yogi merged into the face of a black phallic obelisk from outer space, the yogi is sitting serenely in lotus with an erect penis rising up between his folded legs while his cupped hands, resting on his knees, hold forth the symbols of male and female fertility.

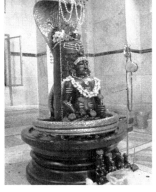

Lord Lakulish on the altar of the Temple of Kayavarohan

Our entourage, including Yogi Desai, arrived in Kayavarohan right after the celebration of Shiva Ratri, the largest holiday on the Indian calendar. It's only equivalent in the U.S. and the West, would be New Year's Eve, where revelry and complete intoxication are precursors for beginning a new year, a new cycle of life, a new you, a new whatever...

We had spent Shiva Ratri the week before at the Temple of

Malav. The towers and steeples of the Temple at Malav boom up from the flat rustic rural landscape like something from another world, or the land of Oz.

During the day of Shiva Ratri, I accompanied Malay Desai on a Jeep ride to see and video what was going on at the more modest local Shiva worship sites. Ancient stone temples housed aged mendicants offering visitors sweets. Outside the temples, there were scores of mopeds and motorcycles that transported whole families (on one cycle) as well as groups of teenagers.

When we returned to the Temple of Malav for the nightly celebration, many of the locals we saw earlier at other sites showed up (mostly the young), though many of the older residents stayed away, perhaps feeling intimidated by the size and grandeur of the new and lavish Temple.

Possibly in deference to its Western guests, the Temple put on a magnificent 4th of July style fireworks show. The locals of course loved it, and we, just as naturally, wanting something more Indian, were somewhat disappointed.

We didn't arrive at Kayavarohan until after the Shiva Ratri celebrations had expired. The Temple in Kayavarohan, with Lord Lakulish ensconced in it in his serenely virile glory is, of course, the main site of worship and celebration during Shiva Ratri. The celebrations last a week and draw hundreds of thousands of people from all over the world – hounds of god, anchorites, every variety of mystic imaginable, old and new school hippies, jetsetters and celebrities.

It was into such a similarly heady and festive atmosphere that Yogi Desai, in 1974, led sixty of his Western disciples into Kayavarohan to celebrate the completed restoration of its resilient and perennially enigmatic 3500 year old temple.

A Fateful Trip

During the three-week stay, as Yogi Desai described it to me, during his three week stay, within the charged atmosphere of day and night-long Shiva Ratri celebrations, he felt pressured by his Indian peers and gave in to overt sexual advances directed towards him by one of his female American disciples. After doing so, he returned home to the United States and to his family and community. The woman, returned to her husband (who had stayed behind to help administer the *ashram*). No one would say mum about the incident for another ten years, at which time Yogi Desai would deny the woman's openly expressed charges. Although by this time she had already separated from her husband, for a variety of other issues, when she was banished from the *ashram* for 'making up lies about the guru', she also lost contact with her former husband and son for an extended period of time.

When I asked Yogi Desai why he did not simply tell the truth about what happened, he answered: "Because I was afraid to. I was afraid of losing everything – my family, the *ashram*. I even thought they might accuse me of rape, which was definitely not what happened, though that charge had been made against others in my position." When I questioned him further about how he felt about doing that, lying, he answered: "I was a human being going through the things a human being goes through, including making mistakes."

The lie would fester for another ten years, until, in Yogi Desai's words: "Reality is relentless. It follows behind every denial, every avoidance, every lie, until it is embraced with open arms."

Amen.

CHAPTER 7:

GRACE TRANSFORMS

'Life is a perpetually therapeutic irritant.'
—Yogi Desai (A lot lately)

I n regards to what happened at Kayavarohan in 1974, and other purported incidents involving Yogi Desai and female disciples, I would like to say that I take Yogi Desai at face value when he says that he was a human being going through the things a human being does, including making mistakes. I'm not saying this to justify his actions or deny his wrongdoing. Being in a position of power and authority, exploiting it, and then securing one's own situation at the emotional and psychological expense of anyone else is, and especially for someone in a position of revered authority, inexcusable.

But I have known Amrit Desai, the person, before, during the crisis, and afterward, and I am firmly convinced that he is someone who is uncommonly dedicated to using his experiences, good or bad, to the best of his ability as a means of transforming his nature for the better.

How?

"The Purpose of my Life is Transformation..."

One day in 1983, at the Kripalu Center in Massachusetts, following a morning of working on *Kripalu Yoga: Meditation in Motion*, Yogi Desai and I got into his car, a white Cadillac, and drove toward Lake Mahkeenac for a mid-day swim. The large beautiful lake, that formed over the ages in a bowl between two long rangy hills on either side of the Center, was a favorite place for residents, guests, and guru alike to enjoy swimming and sailing.

On the way, we stopped by the Kripalu Center to pick up someone who asked to join us. We waited in the main lobby, where there is a floor-to-ceiling wall of glass offering an expansive view of the valley and lake below.

All around the lobby, there were guests and residents busily going about attending to their daily chores and programs. Behind us, there was a gift shop filled with people buying books, tapes, souvenirs and accessories.

Yogi Desai looked out the window and raised his arms. Looking out expansively and somewhat mirthful, he told me: "Look at all this. And it all came about simply because I wanted to create a place to practice and teach yoga and have people around me who also wanted to live a healthy, positive lifestyle."

In *Working Miracles of Love*, Yogi Desai elaborated on those thoughts and feelings more formally: "The purpose for which I was born was transformation – the removal from my consciousness of every limiting concept, emotional block, or thought that separates me from my true self and therefore from God. I have not forced or willed any of my external achievements to happen; rather, they have all occurred naturally as I followed my inner longing for transformation. I have simply responded to what presented itself to me, day by day, and used every situation for my growth. As I have done that, Kripalu has grown and flourished organically."

Because Yogi Desai's self-proclaimed purpose in life is transformation, and not just to practice and teach yoga, the yoga he would develop, as well as the community that would form around him, would likewise conform to this purpose and be dedicated to espousing and serving it.

While Yogi Desai was in seclusion in the early part of 1974, he wrote the following to the Kripalu community: "My love is equally available to all of you. I love each one of you. Each of you is a link in a chain. This chain, which is my support in my deep climbing, is no stronger than its weakest link. It is the duty of each one of you to take every opportunity to help your brother and sister who is in need and keep the chain strong and together through love and service to each other. Once you have come to me and have become a link in the chain, it automatically becomes my responsibility as well as that of the other links to see to the well-being and strength of each link. Your strength is your peace and love; preserve and help reserve it at all times."

For the next twenty years, Yogi Desai's dedication to his *sadhana*, and the unconditional support he receives from his disciples, would become the central force in the dynamic transformation of the Kripalu community from a small rural spiritual commune to the largest and most successful yoga-based enterprise of its kind.

What Makes A Yoga Transformational?

Yogi Desai's promise to himself and his disciples is that together they would embark on a transformational spiritual journey, not just be entrepreneurial pioneers in an alternative business enterprise featuring yoga.

Fundamentally, personal and spiritual transformation through the practice of yoga begins by using the body as a template for recognizing physical, emotional and psychological limitations; and through the confidence-building process of overcoming them, optimize the functioning of one's body, mind and psyche. Optimal functioning, however, is not the be all and end all of the process in transformational yoga, as it is in some physically oriented practices. For a practice of yoga to be transformational, it must make optimal functioning the starting point and foundation for opening a person up to more subtle mental and physical attributes, via practices such as meditation and *pranayamas*. Included among these more subtle and dormant attributes, but not limited to them, are increased intuition, self-direction, peace-of-mind, empathy, and compassion.

One of the innovative and appealing qualities of the practice of Kripalu Yoga is that yoga postures are performed simultaneously with meditation and *pranayamas*. This distinction gives the practice an immediately rewarding and enticing transformational quality for those who are attracted to the practice of yoga for such purpose.

This innovation came as a direct result of Yogi Desai's break-through experience while practicing a conventional routine of yoga postures. When he went into meditation spontaneously while performing the postures he discovered that the life force, or *prana*, could act either mechanically, through the will, or it could act on its own, intuitively. Furthermore, he observed that when it acted mechanically, it often did not act in the body's or the person's best interest. He experimented and determined that this phenomenon of being locked into set, mechanical patterns in yoga, and in life, was often due to emotional, psychological, or physical charges or traumas that happened in the past. He also found that by entering into yoga postures in a meditative state, one could explore these areas of charge, become aware of the relation between mechanical physical movements and psychological and emotional blockages, and, on one's own, work through them.

In a book called *Waking: A Memoir of Trauma and Transcendence* (Rodale Press, 2006), the author, Mathew Sanford, who was paralyzed from the chest down following a car accident at the age of thirteen, relates how he used yoga to explore and overcome trauma. "As I did more and more [yoga] poses, especially twists and backbends, the energy trapped in my spine began to release. As this happened, I would revisit my traumatic past and, in particular, the accident scene. Although difficult in the moment, these experiences catalyzed a new sense of freedom. Finally, the trauma that had struck through my thirteen-year-old body was coming into my field of vision. I was surrounding it. It was no longer surrounding me." Today, Mathew Sanford is married with two children and heads a nonprofit organization called Mind Body Solutions.

In *Kripalu Yoga: Mediation in Motion*, Yogi Desai described some of the ways in which less dramatic psychological and emotional charge can become harmfully settled in the body. "When our actions are in conflict with the body's needs, and repeated habitually, they create chronic stress patterns in the body. The body then begins to deteriorate in those places and we become susceptible to pain and disease. The stress becomes localized in the body into what I call 'energy blocks', which continually sap our vital energy. The purpose of Kripalu Yoga is to remove the physical blocks that continually drain the energy and prevent the free, healing flow of *prana*, and to establish a healthy lifestyle to root out the habitual causes of stress and disease."

One of the most significant contributions Kripalu Yoga is making to the understanding and improvement of the human condition is the focus on the body as a depository for chronic psychological and emotional pain, as well as a vehicle for removing it. The Western approach to deal with these energy blocks has been, until recently, simply to identify them as neurotic. There was no remedy available for the condition other than endlessly talking about it. "Sigmund Freud hardly scratched the surface of human psychology with his investigations. He worked primarily with abnormal psychology, but in truth every human being, so long as he lives in delusion, is a mass of conflicting qualities, or complexes. Freud saw only the conflict between personal desire and the expectations of society. In reality, the case is infinitely more complex." (Paramhansa Yogananda: *The Essence of the Bhagavad Gita*. Crystal Clarity Publishers, 2006.)

In order for the practice of yoga to be transformational, it therefore not only requires a disciplined and focused approach to the practice, but a commitment to making substantial changes to one's physical and emotional condition, as well as one's outlook and lifestyle. Residents joining the Kripalu Ashram at this time committed to living a lifestyle that was quite unorthodox for the average American: to live without personal possessions, or work for an income, and to forgo intimate relationships outside of marriage for at least four years. This was a tremendous adjustment for a twenty- or thirty-year-old to make, especially to a practice and spiritual philosophy that was still largely unknown to most Americans (including resident's families).

People generally do not do something for nothing, and that also includes members of spiritual communities. What the Kripalu community members were banking on is that what they were sacrificing, personally and materially, would be more than made for up by what they'd gain in other ways: to live and work in a safe, secure and relatively stress-free environment; to eat nutritious, well-balanced meals prepared daily; and, last but not least, an opportunity to learn yoga – its philosophy and practice – directly from a Yogi.

In order for the exchange to work, and not simply create material and personal ennui and conflicts, a bond of trust had to be established between Yogi Desai and the leaders of the Kripalu community and its residential staff, that ensured each that they were integral parts of a graceful journey called *sadhana* that would take them to the highest levels of yoga (and human potential). Within the Kripalu community, there was always a percentage of residents who were content to be there just to live in a beautiful setting without the usual stresses they previously experienced working regular jobs. Though there were a significant number of residents who wanted, and expected, more. And the 'more' that they were seeking was personal and spiritual transformation.

The Secret Ingredient in Grace that Transforms: Shaktipat Kundalini

"Only that person who knows *Kundalini* knows Yoga." Shrii Kripalvanandji. (*The Stages of Kundalini Yoga*, Kripalu Publications, 1975.)

If we accept that animate life is animated by something, and that humans are animate, than there must be some force that animates us. In yogic philosophy, as well as other spiritual traditions, this animating force is believed to be breath, oxygen, or *prana*.

Prana is the Sanskrit term for breath, life-force and spirit. Some of the 'secret' or esoteric practices that Swami Chandra imparted to Amrit Desai as a youth included various *pranayamas*, techniques for controlling the breath and at the same time purifying and exulting the mind and body. The willful control and manipulation of breath is vital in yoga and meditation, as it is synonymous with the two-fold essential purpose of yoga: quieting the incessant fluctuations of the mind, and purifying as well as nurturing and optimizing the life force or spirit. Combining the practice of yoga postures, which opens the body to allow in greater and greater amounts of life-force, with the practice of *pranayama* that helps flatten the mind's undulations, often induces temporary altered states of consciousness, such as *samadhi*.

That is why, in the early stages of *Shaktipat Kundalini* Yoga, initial experiences of spiritual awakening are described as '*prana* awakenings.' Though, as Shrii Kripalvanandji points out: "The rousing of *Prana* is different from the awakening of *Kundalini*. Aroused *Prana* does not penetrate the *Chakras* (nerve centers) and

Granthis (plexuses), nor does it completely purify the body and mind. This task is performed only when the Kundalini power is awakened through the rousing of *Prana*. To awaken Kundalini is one thing and to make it move upward is another thing."

The difference between 'aroused' *prana* and mundane *prana* is that the latter happens without our conscious involvement. When we are asleep or under an anesthetic, for instance, the lungs continue to ventilate oxygen throughout the body, maintaining metabolic functioning with or without our willful cooperation. When one consciously 'super-animates' the body by intentionally increasing one's capacity to take in, manipulate, sublimate and discharge the invisible forces animated by *prana*, through practices such as meditation and *pranayama*, the process initiates changes within the human body and mind on a par – though more sublime –with the external discharge of energy via the intentional manipulation of invisible entities such as atoms. No one has yet seen an atom, though no one doubts their existence and potential power. No one also has ever seen a *prana*, or the 'dark' matter that permeates the universe. So be it; these invisible forces are all around and in us, waiting to reveal ever more exotic qualities, powers and surprises.

In his book, *Spiritual Nutrition* (North Atlantic Books, 2005), Gabriel Cousins, who received *Shaktipat Diksha* from the Indian Yogi, Swami Muktananda, described *Kundalini* awakening this way: "*Kundalini* is the inner spiritualizing energy that takes us to the experience of noncausal ecstasy, joy, peace, love, and God awareness. *Kundalini* is the Grace of God."

Gopi Krishna, another renowned India Yogi, who had a *Kundalini* awakening experience in 1937, wrote about it lucidly in

Kundalini: Path to Higher Consciousness (Orient Paperbacks, New Delhi 1992). He described the implications of his experience as such: "A new center presently dormant in the average man and woman has to be activated and a more powerful stream of psychic energy must stream forth to the head from the base of the spine to allow human consciousness to transcend the human limits. This is the final phase of the present evolutionary impulse in man."

And, finally, the modern Western psychologist Carl Jung offered this perspective: 'When you succeed in awakening the *Kundalini*, so that it starts to move out of its mere potentiality, you necessarily start a world that is totally different from our world. It is the world of eternity." (*Psychological Commentary on Kundalini Yoga*, New York, Spring Publications, 1975).

There are traditionally two distinct paths within the formal practice and dissemination of this advanced form of yoga. In *The Stages of Kundalini* Yoga, Shrii Kripalvanandji described it this way: "There are two types of devotion, one believing in knowledge and one believing in action. Therefore, although there is but one yoga, it has two states, *Gnana* Yoga and *Karma* Yoga. In *Gnana* Yoga, the quality of self-mastery being prominent, *Gnana* (knowledge) is given importance, while in *Karma* Yoga, the quality of service being prominent, *Karma* (action), is given importance."

The emphasis on and development of the former practice is what distinguishes yoga from other spiritual practices. Catholics have cloistered monks, as do Buddhists. They live their lives in pacific seclusion and pray that they may have some subtle and noble prophylactic effect on saving the human race from completely destroying itself. The Yogi, or *Shakti* Guru, however, dynamically

channels and disseminates spiritual knowledge, energy and experience via esoteric practices and non-verbal transmissions. When
Lord Krishna and his disciple, Arjuna, go into battle against the
human forces of delusion and evil in the *Mahabharata*, they are
not there just to observe or settle for a draw, or make a compromise.
They are there to annihilate those negative attributes by overpowering
them with higher-consciousness.

Because this is a task that requires tremendous drive, knowledge,
endurance and determination, the yogi must first prepare himself.
Individual yoga, practiced under the guidance or inspiration of a
self-realized person, or *guru*, is where yogis venture into the
furthermost realms of human potential and experience – seeking
levels of empirical knowledge and dynamic spiritual force that will
first of all allow them to become liberated from the tyrannical grip
of the unconscious and subconscious, and then pass on this
knowledge and experience to others. "Self-realization and the
knowledge of God are synonymous." (Paramahansa Yogananda,
The Essence of the Bhagavad Gita, California, Crystal Clarity
Publications, 2006).

Social yoga is as equally and symbiotically important as
individual yoga, because it is one of the civilizing influences that
keeps societies, families and nations on a high enough keel to
support the adventures of yogis. (In this sense, Indian social yoga
with its network of *ashrams*, holy sites and its public support for
peripatetic holy men and women, is not that different from the
more formal Western philanthropic institutions that finance,
support and maintain the work of scientists, academics and artists.)

Shrii Kripalvanandji clearly chose the path of *Gnana* Yoga and self-mastery and has been recognized around the world for his personal accomplishments as a yogi, as well as venerated for his contributions to literature, music and human society at large. In his lifetime, even though he lived sequestered for twenty-five years while practicing a ten-hour-a-day *Kundalini Shaktipat* Yoga *sadhana*, he restored a Temple, raised the funds to provide education and health care for tens of thousands of Indian children, inspired the discovery of a new form of yoga in America and founded of the largest Center for Yoga and Health in America.

The faith of the yogi acting alone is that the gains they make in their personal spiritual practice will not only have subtle effects, but will also directly and dramatically change and enhance the quality of life around them.

An Artistic and, of Course, Precarious New Path

Yogi Desai, on the other hand, like the Yoga he discovered, attempted to combine the two states of yoga into one practice. A practitioner of Kripalu Yoga is not only afforded the possibility of accessing the deepest levels of *Kundalini Shaktipat* yoga, but is also allowed, or mandated by example, to stay 'in motion' or in the world, while doing so.

In Chapter 2 of this book, I described how Amrit Desai came to the United States to study art and then chose teaching yoga because, in his words, it was "the bigger canvas." Although Yogi Desai stopped operating in a particular form of art, it seems obvious that he did not stop being an artist. It's his artistic predisposition to take what's given and create something new from it that makes him choose, time and again, the roads less visited.

In his lifetime, Yogi Desai will reap both fantastic rewards for his maverick innovations, as well as pay a very steep price for them, nearly losing everything he worked his life for. "For this journey contains innumerable twists and turns. There is but one guideline that can give it right direction: The polestar of one's innate divinity." (Paramahansa Yogananda, *The Essence of the Bhagavad Gita*, Crystal Clarity Publications, California, 2006).

As Grace and *Shakti* continue to twist and turn, transforming those who are open to it in the ways that it, and they will, Yogi Amrit Desai and the Kripalu community soon get an unexpected and welcomed gift of Grace – a visit from a living polestar of innate divinity.

CHAPTER 8:

(INFINITY) LIVING GRACE

Shrii Kripalvanandji Visits and then Resides in America

Whenever Yogi Desai visited India he tried to entice Shrii Kripalvanandji to come and visit his new community of American disciples at the Kripalu Ashram in Pennsylvania.

It had always felt – to Yogi Desai and the Kripalu community – like a long shot.

First of all, as I noted in previous chapters, Shrii Kripalvanandji was engaged in a daily and all-encompassing *Kundalini* Yoga *sadhana*. In addition to that, he was the head, or spiritual director, of the Temple of Kayavarohan, one of the major and busiest spiritual sites in India. When he was not in *sadhana*, while still maintaining silence, he wrote written guidance, giving specific instructions for the administration of the Temple, as well as its humanitarian projects. Overall, his attention was distracted from his *sadhana*, by the mundane activities of directing a Temple.

Yogi Desai's most appealing, and in the end, winning offer to Shrii Kriplvanandji, was that if he came to America, he would not have any bureaucratic responsibilities, social activities, or personal obligations. He could focus exclusively on his *sadhana* in the private, isolated residence the Kripalu community had built for Yogi Desai when he went into seclusion, *Muktidam*.

During a visit by Yogi Desai to India in the winter of 1977, Shrii Kripalvanandji gazed at Yogi Desai and spoke in a hushed tone: "Today I have good news for you. I will come to America. But remember, I am not coming as a missionary, to change people, or to spread my teachings. I am not coming for money or fame, or to increase my circle of disciples. I am not coming to be with my spiritual grandchildren. I'm coming because of your love." (*The Life of Yogi Amrit Desai,* Kripalu Publications, 1982.)

Ecstatic, Yogi Desai immediately called the Kripalu Ashram in the middle of the night with the news that Shrii Kripalvanandji would be coming to America in three months time, during summer.

The immediate reaction of the community was one of disbelief and incredulousness. How many times previously had their hopes been hyped then diminished. At this point their namesake was more of an apparition than a concrete reality.

So Yogi Desai returned to the United States a few months in advance of Shrii Kripalvanandji's arrival in order to prepare the residents of the *ashram* for accepting, welcoming and experiencing him. Yogi Desai vehemently instructed them to intensify their personal yoga *sadhana*, especially the practices of meditation, *pranayama* and *mantra*.

Yogi Desai explained: "Bapuji (Shrii Kripalvanandji) is such a

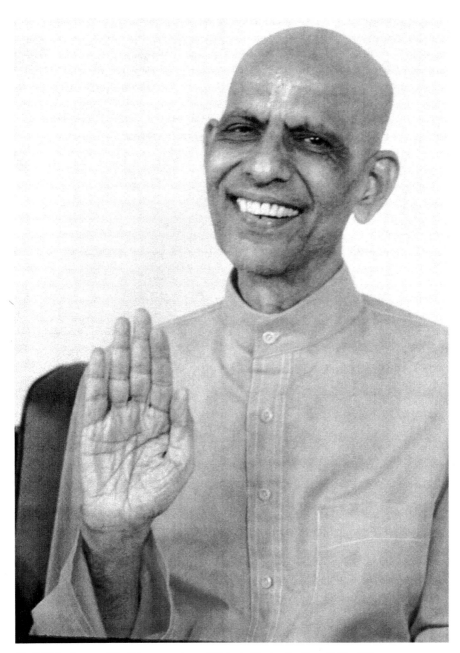

Shrii Kripalvanandji   *(Photo courtesy of Kripalu Center for Yoga & Health)*

being that it is very difficult for the mind, or the usual consciousness, to comprehend his magnitude. Externally, he appears to lead a regular life. He eats ordinary food and when necessary, he discusses administrative matters related to his humanitarian work in India. Yet he is a saint. He is one of the greatest living masters on this earth. Everyone feels that about their *guru*, but Bapuji has demonstrated this. He has shown an exquisite degree of tolerance, patience, and perseverance in his search for God. He has meditated for ten hours a day for twenty-five years, and has maintained complete silence for twelve of those years. Since 1971, he has spoken only on rare occasions when he addressed large groups during sacred celebrations. Our ability to experience Bapuji is directly proportional to the teachings that we have digested. I want each one of you to increase your capacity to absorb our master while he is with us. Nothing is more powerful for increasing your capacity than love. What do I mean when I say 'love'? Love means total openness and receptivity, without imposing any of your expectations. To receive from a master you must be totally still inside. If you meet Bapuji with tension and expectations, you will not meet the master; Bapuji will disappear. To go for the *darshan* (be in the presence) of a saint or master, you must go empty and humbly, so that he may fill you up. If received properly, Bapuji can transform your life. You all must have truly prayed for Bapuji's visit. No one in India could actually believe that he is coming. This is the wonder that love can perform."

Yogi Desai then returned to India in order to join an entourage that accompanied Shrii Kripalvanandji to America. At New York's J.F.K. airport, he was welcomed in the diplomatic lounge reserved for arriving dignitaries. Hundreds of Shrii Kripalvanandji's disciples from throughout North America were there to greet him.

As he sat in the diplomatic lounge, in lotus, smiling blissfully, Shrii Kripalvanandji wrote down his thoughts and feelings and Yogi Desai translated them aloud: "My beloved children, there was absolutely no possibility of my coming to America. And yet, I have come, drawn by your pure love. It is well known that a magnet has the power to attract iron. You are all magnets of love, and you have attracted me here. I have not come here to propagate yoga, or meditation or religion. I have simply come to greet you. What an amazing happening this is. Where is India, where is America. Truly, love knows no distinction between countries, dress, appearance, virtue, age. I have a firm and complete faith that your pure love will be of great help to me in completing my *sadhana*. As your spiritual grandfather, my blessing is that this entire group of

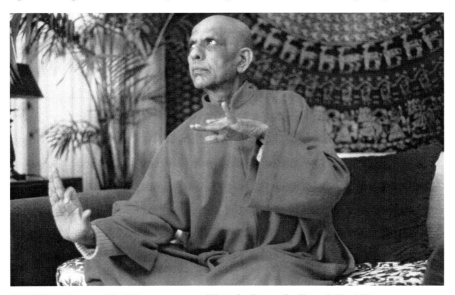

Shrii Kripalvanandji   *(Photo courtesy of Kripalu Center for Yoga & Health)*

seekers may go all the way to the gates of God."

Shrii Kripalvanandji and Yogi Desai drove back to the Kripalu
Ashram in Sumneytown where Shrii Kripalvanandji, as promised,
took up residence in *Muktidham*.

During the first five months of his planned nine-month visit, he
was very generous with his time and conducted daily 6 A.M. *satsangas*
with residents and guests of the *ashram* and mid-afternoon *darshans*
on Sundays.

Following the five-month period of being available publicly,
Shrii Kripalvanandji returned to seclusion and *sadhana*, giving
only two public discourses a year during the remainder of his
unexpected and welcomed four-and-a-half-year stay in *Muktidham*.
The following are some excerpts from those discourses (taken
from *Pilgrimage of Love*, Book II, Kripalu Publications, 1984):

On Dharma (Social Yoga):

"When human beings were first born on earth, everyday living
was filled with complicated problems. For many ages, man struggled
just to survive. At last he was able to try to make his existence a
happy one. He established the family, society and a nation to form
a system of life: *dharma*. Man had suffered for many years due to a
lack of *dharma*; so he set forth *dharma* in order to acquire peace,
happiness and bliss. One who does not understand *dharma* does
not understand life. *Dharma* is the pilgrimage of life and cannot be
separated from it. In fact, a concept of *dharma* that is separate from
life cannot be called *dharma*. The attribute that makes humans
special is *dharma*."

On Knowledge:

"Ignorance is *adharma*: it brings unhappiness to each and every human being. Bondage is the result of ignorance. Knowledge is *dharma*, which results in happiness for each and every individual. Liberation is the result of knowledge. Adherence to *dharma* causes evolution of the mind; adherence to *adharma* causes distortion of the mind. That which liberates from bondage is knowledge. Knowledge is what allows one to cross over inertia and beastliness and attain humanity and divinity. In modern times, knowledge is defined as that which results in fame and wealth. Until there is a change in the definition of knowledge, there will be no change in the direction of individuals, families, societies, or nations. In order to create unity, one must live a life that expresses love for family, society and nation. Until we think of others in our family, society and nation, we must be considered adharmic, uncultured and inhuman."

[For ages in India, yoga was a communal activity, practiced collectively in order to create a viable and tenable social structure or *dharma*. The collective elevation of the mind and emotions that accompanies the practice of good *dharma* in time brought about the spiritual philosophy and science that became Hinduism. It also allowed individuals to venture outside the worldly planes in order to discover forms of esoteric knowledge and realization.]

Distinction between Worldly and Heavenly Dharma:

"*Pravritti dharma* is the family *dharma*, social *dharma* and national *dharma*. It appears to be an ordinary religion. On the contrary, if it were ordinary, it would have been practiced from the beginning. The fact that *pravritti dharma* took many centuries to be established proves that it is extraordinary. Love, surrender and service are the foremost aspects of *dharma*. Aversion, greed and tyranny are the foremost aspects of *adharma*. People can become followers of any religious sect; this is their right and should not be opposed. However, the *dharma* that each person has in him does not become effective until he practices it in everyday life. The world appears hungry and thirsty because *dharma* is not practiced in life. People have learned *pravritti dharma* from their *guru*, and this agrees with their internal sense of *dharma*; however they have not practiced it. When one aspires to *nivritti dharma*, which is meant for greatmasters, one is trying to jump from earth to reach the holy feet of Almighty God. However, he does not realize that if he does not succeed at *pravritti dharma*, he does not deserve *nivritti dharma*.

On Yogi Desai and Kripalu Yoga:

"The *sadhana* of *prana* is *nivritti dharma*, and the *sadhana* of *chitta* (mindstuff) is *pravritti dharma*. *Nivritti dharma* is for the great master who is a genuine seeker of liberation. The *sadhak* (practitioner) of *pravritti dharma*, who desires wealth, passion and *dharma* gives up *prana* and takes the help of *chitta*. *Pravritti dharma* is the *dharma* of family, society and nation. It is useful to all. I first taught the *sadhana* of *chitta* to Amrit Desai. Through this he has attained success according to his desires. For this reason he has experienced the *sadhana* of *chitta* as being the one best for him, giving him love and faith. His followers have also had the same experience. Because of this success, he has called this *chitta sadhana* 'Kripalu Yoga' and has spread it everywhere."

On Life & Struggle:

"The life of every individual is indeed 'life', but each individual's life differs according to its special aim. Thus, it is difficult to give a definition of life that includes everyone. Life has two currents: the flow of happiness and the flow of unhappiness. Because of this, we can make several definitions of life. Life is an endless circle of mistakes which can never be prevented. Life is a chaotic mixture of happiness and unhappiness. Life means struggle. All these definitions connote unhappiness. All these definitions are perfect, yet imperfect. If on the other hand, we look at a definition of life that connotes happiness; then life means love; life means progress; life means light; life means evolutions; and life means happiness, peace, bliss. These definitions, however, are very ordinary because they convey only a vague conception and understanding of life. The second word to consider is struggle. Struggle means competition, malice and rivalry for battle. Here we will take the definition of struggle as 'battle' only, because clash, competition, rivalry and malice are all encompassed by the word 'battle'. This world is a battlefield. Anyone who is born has to be a warrior. Whether one is a boy or a girl, man or women, young or old, king or beggar, brave or cowardly, literate or illiterate, saint or sinner, he has to fight the battle. Without fighting the battle, self-protection is impossible. The major duty (*dharma*) in this world is to fight. There are numerous kinds of battles and warriors. Battles begin with birth and exist up to the last breath of life. Life can end, but the battle cannot... Even very wise men create huge forts to prevent struggle from entering their lives, but it enters nonetheless. Struggle is the *prana* of every person's life. Struggle guides everyone's life. Struggle leads human beings from untruth to truth, from ignorance to knowledge, from darkness to light, and from death to immortality. Struggle is everyone's friend. It is proper to welcome struggle. Its arrival is always auspicious. It is such a noble door that it never asks the recipient to come to it. It goes to the door of the individual, gives whatever it wants to give, gives it privately, and walks away silently. Struggle is a very skillful sculptor. It creates a very beautiful idol from an ugly rock. It changes the sub-human into an ideal human being and transforms an ordinary human being into a *deva* (human deity) who is respected by the whole world. Struggle is a subtle sculptor who shapes the life of every great master of the world into a unique and unparalleled work of art."

On Celibacy:

"Celibacy is the major principle at the root of *pravritti dharma* and *nivritti dharma*. In *pravritti dharma*, celibacy is practiced to the best of one's ability. In *nivritti dharma*, the aspirant practices celibacy to become an *urdhvareta* yogi, or perfect celibate, whose sexual fluid is sublimated. Both paths need to be understood perfectly. To be celibate is one thing; to be *urdhvareta* is another. There are two kinds of passion which arise in everyone's body: physical-spiritual and mental-sensual. Physical passion is a result of *prana*. The awakening of passion in a child's body is the result of *prana*; it is not a conscious phenomenon; The sexual center in the *chitta,* or mindstuff, of the child is undeveloped; therefore passion is not produced there. If there is any passion at all, it is in a very subtle form and the child is not conscious of it. The passion born of *prana* is described as spiritual, because through it a yogi becomes *urdhvareta.* When in *sahaj* (spontaneous, meditative) yoga the independent *prana* awakens the sleeping *kundalini* energy through the pressure of the heel of the foot in the perineum (the area between the anus and the posterior part of the external genitalia; from the Sanskrit 'to set in motion'), then spiritual passion is born. In both the *pravritti* and *nivritti dharmas,* it is necessary to awaken the *kundalini shakti;* otherwise there is no possibility of any attainment. The *kundalini* awakens in a minute and tolerable form in all the techniques of *pravritti dharma;* however, the steadiness of the *sadhak 's chitta* is not disturbed. In *nivritti dharma,* all the techniques used to awaken the *kundalini shakti* awaken it in its complete, intolerable and terrifying form, and the *sadhak* is unable to protect the steadiness of the *chitta* because of the strength of the *prana.* To maintain steadiness of mind, the true seeker of liberation retires from worldly contact and activity and observes seclusion. The path of the yogi is not nearly as easy as that of the child, because the sexual center in the yogi's *chitta* is fully developed, and passion is produced there. The passion produced by *chitta* and the passion produced by *kundalini* become one; this becomes an obstacle in the path of the yogi. This is such an overwhelmingly difficult stage that only a perfect yogi can give true guidance to a *sadhak* faced with it. No one else can give this guidance. Others who give guidance at this stage do so from logic and not from experience."

Shrii Kripalvanandji, like his protégé, Yogi Desai, had an artistic temperament. His artistic expression manifested itself through storytelling. Here is one such example from Shrii Kripalvanandji's *Pilgrimage of Love*, Volume I, Kripalu Publications, 1982.

Anecdote: Vasavdatta meets Upgupatta:

Vasavdatta was a very beautiful prostitute. She entertained aristocrats at her magnificent residence or sometimes at their palatial homes.

One enchanting full moon night, Vasavdatta was engrossed in beautifying her body. She wore make-up, sensuous clothing, and jewelry. Finally, she adorned her hair with fragrant flowers and sprayed expensive perfume on her sari dress. The house became pervaded with a sweet fragrance.

It was time to leave. In the courtyard, the charioteer stood waiting in his chariot. Feeling delighted, Vasavdatta seated herself in the chariot and directed the charioteer, "Sumantra, this is a radiant full-moon night. Drive along the lakeshore so we can enjoy its natural beauty."

She was going as a beloved to an appointment made by her lover, and her heart was blooming like a thousand petaled lotus. Her lover's home was in a secluded spot near the lake. As the chariot moved and they approached the lake, her eyes suddenly came to rest upon a figure on the lakeshore.

There sat a Buddhist monk, Upgupatta, meditating with closed eyes. Radiant with the splendor of celibacy, his body glistened in the moonlight. Vasavdatta had never seen such a beautiful sight. She completely forgot the lover she had originally set out to meet.

(Was he then her lover? No, for if he were truly her beloved, she could not have forgotten him in such a flash.) She was a prostitute with innumerable lovers, each with eyes thirsty for beauty and passion. How could pure love reside there?

Vasavdatta halted the chariot close to the shore. Quietly alighting, she approached Upgupatta. Her jingling anklets caught his attention, and he opened his eyes. Although he beheld a celestial damsel standing before him, Upgupatta was not influenced by her arrival or by her beauty. Vasavdatta peered into his crystal clear eyes, which contained neither passion nor the desire for beauty. Never in her life had she seen such a pure and wholesome gaze.

At that moment, her Indian heritage reflected back to her thought, 'He is a saint. His body and mind are very pure. It is a great sin to look at him with passionate eyes.'

Yet, this thought did not remain in her mind for long. Vasavdatta had mastered the art of overwhelming her lovers with passion, but now she found herself completely helpless for the first time. Was the thirst for pure love awakening in her?

While drinking in the nectar of his beauty, Vasavdatta found herself gently praying to him, "Oh Divine One! I have accidentally come upon your feet, and in a mere moment I have become yours. Kindly accept me. I humbly beg for your love."

Hearing her request, neither his eyes nor his speech reflected anger or humiliation. Rather, Upgupatta's eyes were flooded with pure love as he replied, "Divine lady, right now I am meditating; let me continue and tomorrow I will come to your home."

Astonished, she inquired, "You'll come to my home?"

"Of course," he replied.

"Your Holiness, do you know who I am?" Vasavdatta asked timidly.

"No, I do not know who you are."

"I am Vasavdatta, a well-known prostitute in this city."

"Where do you live?" came the unconcerned voice of the saint.

"Near the Devkunj."

"All right, then, that is where I will meet you," he said agreeably.

She continued to gaze at him for some time without batting an eyelash, and finally asked, "Wouldn't you hesitate to come there?"

"Where is there hesitancy in love?" he firmly replied. The word 'love' resounded in her ears like the sweet strumming of a stringed instrument. Her mind was exalted. Longing to hear it again, Vasavdatta exclaimed, "Do you love me?"

With sublime steadiness, the saint replied, "A few moments ago, you yourself begged me for love."

Again, Vasavdatta experienced a tender joy and immediately felt awkward. Excusing herself, she said, "I do not want to distract your meditation. I will await you tomorrow at lunchtime."

With that, Upgupatta immediately closed his eyes and continued meditating. Meanwhile, Vasavdatta seated herself in her chariot and directed the charioteer to take her back home.

Over the past few years, Vasavdatta had been playing the game of love. But today the flame of pure love was enkindled of its own accord in the temple of her heart. No longer an erring prostitute, Vasavdatta had now become a pure adolescent. Mentally she had married her chosen husband. Although she could not imagine how long this marriage would last, she smiled radiantly. *She felt that her few moments of exquisite pure love had far surpassed her years spent in passionate pursuits. No woman becomes a prostitute of her own accord. Helplessness makes her a prostitute. The eternal qualities of pure love do not leave her even if she is a prostitute. Rather, this pure love lies dormant and determined in her heart.*

The next day was auspicious in every way. Vasavdatta carefully bathed and dressed herself in white clothing. Someone unfamiliar with her would have guessed that she was an ascetic from the forest visiting the city. She and her maidservants began transforming her home, removing expensive sensual material from the dining room and replacing it with only a modest carpet. Next, she went to the kitchen and prepared very simple food. Although Vasavdatta had a treasury of golden serving ware, she asked the servants to bring plantain leaves for dishes. *'How could man-made utensils compare with the sublime beauty of God's creation?'*

Vasavdatta finished all her arrangements and eagerly awaited Upgupatta in the gallery. When he arrived, Vasavdatta affectionately welcomed him and invited him to dine. Neither spoke during the meal. Upgupatta's eyes were very pleased at the sight of her external changes.

After sitting for some time, he finally excused himself, saying he had to leave.

"You're leaving?" she replied with fright.

"Naturally," he stated. "I came only to offer alms of love. My purpose is finished. Now I must leave."

"So this is love?" she inquired insistently.

"Yes," he replied. "Whatever satisfies the body and mind with a mere drop is called love."

"Your Holiness! But I have not received the satisfaction of which you speak," asserted Vasavdatta.

"That is due to your own lack of penance," replied Upgupatta. *"One cannot attain love without penance. Only after penance purifies the body and mind can the drop of love nectar be secreted. If a mere drop of poison can cause death, then a mere drop of nectar can imbue immortality."*

"But Divine One!" she protested. "Not only do I belong to this mortal world, but I am even more impure and unworthy than an ordinary woman. My only desire in this life is that you might touch me once more."

Upgupatta stood motionless. He closed his eyes for a moment and then promised her, "Divine and fair Lady, I assure you that I will come one day to bless you with a touch. Your penance is to wait until that time. I give my solemn promise."

"I have faith in your word and will await you," she submitted humbly.

As Upgupatta left, Vasavdatta collapsed to the floor.

Several years passed. Stricken with the dreaded disease of syphilis, Vasavdatta began to experience its torment. Her beauty was painfully transformed into ugliness daily as the disease ran its course. At the same time, an epidemic of plague struck the city. Vasavdatta also fell victim to its ravages, and along with others who had become infected, she was cast out of the city into a ditch.

One night, when the full moon spread its light upon her, the unconscious Vasavdatta began coming to her senses. Upon opening her eyes, she experienced great thirst but could not get up. Death was too near. Still, she yearned for a few drops of water to wet her parched throat. Looking around, Vasavdatta saw that there wasn't a living person to be found. Only a few dead bodies lay off in the distance. There was no one to quench the thirst of the woman who used to drink water from a golden cup. Her eyes filled with tears; her only desire was for water and there was nothing she could do!

Suddenly, she heard someone's footsteps. Slowly turning her head in the direction of the sound, Vasavdatta was filled with joy and surprise. Upgupatta was coming. Suddenly, distress ran off into the distance while immense joy came running to her side. Indeed it was he. It was the same body, splendid with the light of celibacy, which she had seen on the lakeshore. Now he was here by her side, just as bright and magnificent as ever. Silently he sat down.

In a barely audible voice Vasavdatta exclaimed, "You did come after all! I am so happy. Now I will die in peace."

As Upgupatta took her head in his lap, Vasavdatta cried out loudly, "No! No! Please don't touch me. My sickness will infect your body!"

Indifferent to her plea, he took her head in his lap and said with utmost love, "Fair Lady! Do not trouble yourself about my body. I promised to give you happiness with my touch. I have come to fulfill my promise."

Vasavdatta's eyes clouded with tears. Innumerable times she had experienced pleasure through the sense of touch; but the happiness of this sensation was beyond comparison. This was the touch of God. Her body, which had once competed with the charm of the moon, was now riddled with syphilis. But here was a new sensation! Where anyone else would have been repulsed, Upgupatta was showering divine love upon her.

As soon as he lifted the vessel of water, she remembered that her throat was parched. She opened her mouth. Experiencing her thirst quenched, Vasavdatta fell into reverie: "Are these drops of water or of love?" The taste was love. As Upgupatta's hand affectionately caressed her head, Vasavdatta was satisfied drinking the nectar of love.

In a few moments, Vasavdatta felt her mind descending into unknown depths. The dark shadow of death was approaching her. Attempting to fold her hands in prayer, she looked up at Upgupatta; and with eyes fading into the darkness she greeted him.

Pray daily to the Lord on a regular basis. Observe celibacy, and seek the company of moderate diet and exercise. Slowly proceed on the pilgrimage of life, carrying the lamp of good conduct in one hand and the lamp of sexual abstinence in the other. My auspicious blessings to you all.

Shrii Kripalvanandji's last Message to his Followers:

September 27,1981

"Beloved children, do not give up virtuous conduct and self-discipline, even in the face of death. Keep unflinching faith in the holy lotus feet of the Lord and continue practicing *mantra, japa, bhajans*, chanting His name, meditation, *pranayama*, postures, observing holy vows, fasting, moderation in diet, studying scriptures and other disciplines. I extend my blessings to everyone."

Your loving Grandfather,
Kripalu

Dharma, Sadhana, and Service Become the Guideposts for The Kripalu Community:

Through the presence, *sadhana* and words of Shrii Kripalvanandji, the Kripalu Ashram became an intentional community devoted to practicing the principles of good *dharma*, *sadhana* and *karma* (service). Shrii Kriplvanandji remained in residence at *Muktidham* until 1981 when he returned to India for his final act of *sadhana*, or *Mahasamadhi*, after which he was entombed into the bowels of the Temple of Malav.

The sublime Grace Shrii Kripalvanandji, brought to America by his empirical understanding of yoga, permeated the lives of Yogi Desai and the Kripalu community and would be the backbone of strength and resiliency. Each would need to survive the growing pains, and the even greater depths of understanding and accomplishment, the potent gift of Activated Grace, *Kundalini Shaktipat*, inevitably brings forth.

CHAPTER 9:

GRACE SQUANDERED

Growing Pains and a Big Time Move

Although the former corporate retreat in Summit Station provided much needed additional housing and office space, along with an excellent opportunity for Kripalu community members to hone their skills as business people, teachers, and service providers, it was located in a part of Pennsylvania that was not welcoming to yoga, yogis, and off-the-grid backpackers trekking in from across the country and around the world. The dynamic young community's opportunities for growth and expansion were severely limited by their location.

When the Kripalu Yoga Fellowship, a non-profit trust created to oversee the business interests of the Kripalu community, learned of the availability of a 350-acre property in the Berkshire Hills of Massachusetts, its CEO, Sandra Healy, drove to Massachusetts where she indefatigably lobbied politicians and business owners to allow the Kripalu Yoga Fellowship to purchase the property and its facilities.

Ms. Healy, who had been a successful businesswoman in California before joining the Kripalu community, had an independent and personal vision for the Kripalu enterprise, and Yogi Desai, that far outreached what most of the others in the community could envision (or want). She also felt that she had the insight, skills and experience to elevate the Kripalu enterprise, and Yogi Desai's stature, if given the opportunity.

This was her chance and she went for it with a characteristically single-minded gusto.

There were several favorable factors already in place before Ms. Healy's arrival to lobby for a Kripalu Yoga Retreat in the Berkshires. One, was that there was a huge acreage of property – uninhabited and unattended for a decade – that had gone to seed. Its building facilities – a former Jesuit seminary and novitiate – were in a similarly defunct condition as the property.

Overall, the real-estate package had become a white elephant, and, even more importantly, a negative asset to the State. The governor of Massachusetts at the time, Michael Dukakis, proposed using the property to facilitate a minimum-security prison.

Another factor was that the local merchants and business owners, who catered to tourism, expectantly, were vehemently opposed to the idea of placing a prison of any sort in the heart of the Berkshires. These business owners quickly formed a political action lobby group of their own called the Shadowbrook Committee, whose sole purpose was to block the governor's proposal. Ms. Healy no doubt noted that the committee was made invincible by the presence on it of the venerable and lucrative Tanglewood

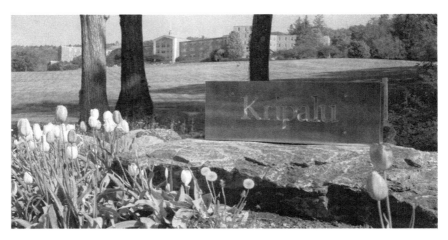

The Kripalu Center for Yoga and Health in Lenox, Massachusetts
(Photo courtesy of Kripalu Center for Yoga & Health)

Music Festival, which was located just a stone's throw from
the property in question.

Another underlying, though very important dynamic in favor of
Ms. Healy's proposition, was that the Kripalu Yoga Fellowship and
the Kripalu community and Retreat in Pennsylvania had not only
been in existence for ten years and was solvent, but it also had
been scandal free. Furthermore, the 200 plus population of its
community was made up of the same demographic (young, white,
and middle-class, though coed) that would have been coming to
Shadowbrook a decade earlier in order to become Jesuits. The
final, and probably the most important ingredient, was Ms. Healy
herself. She was energetic, charming, persuasive, intelligent,
worldly, and determined not to take no for an answer. She also had
personal motivations for acquiring the property that transcended,
so to speak, mere ambition for fame and fortune.

In the winter of 1983 – in what was not a unanimous or confident
decision – the Stockbridge city council agreed to allow the Kripalu

Yoga Fellowship to purchase the 350 acres of land and building facilities, as is, for just over $3,000,000.

A Storied Place

The property was poeticized in American literature by the Transcendentalist writer Nathaniel Hawthorne. In the Introductory to *Tanglewood Tales*, he wrote: "They [The Berkshire Hills] are better than mountains, because they do not stamp and stereotype themselves into the brain, and thus grow wearisome with the same strong impression, repeated day after day. A few summer weeks among mountains, a lifetime among green meadows and placid slopes, with outlines forever new, because continually fading out of the memory – such would be my sober choice... on the shore of the lake, in the dell of Shadow Brook, in the playroom, at Tanglewood fireside, and in a magnificent palace of snow, with ice windows...."

Long before Hawthorne's rapturous prose, the original inhabitants of the bowl of land formed by prehistoric volcanic eruptions and glacial deposits had named it, in Mahkeenac dialect, Happy Valley. They were reverent of the tract of land and forbade warfare or settlement on it. It was reserved for summits, treaties and celebrations, shared with egalitarian high-mindedness by the Mahicans, Iroquois and Mohawks. Over eons, a crystal blue lake had formed at the base of this lush, hilly dell that would come to be known as the Stockbridge Bowl. In spring and throughout the summer, ice melting on hilltops feeds the lake with countless streams and brooks. The lake was named for the 'people of the continuous flowing waters', Lake Mahkeenac. It is the largest body of water in the southern extension of the Green Mountains, and sits nine hundred feet above sea level.

After the Indians were cleared out via the federal government's Indian Resettlement Act following the Revolutionary War, the Stockbridge Bowl became a sanctuary and inspiration for many American writers, artists, and musicians, including Norman Rockwell, Herman Melville, Charles Ives, and Edgar Allen Poe.

Though it wouldn't be until the Gilded Age – the turn of the century period of unbridled capitalism and individual wealth creation – when the rustic valley would become widely inhabited again, this time by wealthy industrialists and financiers occupying palatial mansions charily called 'cottages'.

Chief among these was a manor home built by the railroad magnate turned banker, Anson Phelps Stokes. His manor was the largest privately owned home in America at the time, with over 100 rooms on 1,000 acres of hills and dells landscaped by Frederick Law Olmstead, the architect who designed Central Park in Manhattan. Anson Stokes was a literate gentleman, and gilded, so he named his manor Shadowbrook Castle.

Mr. Stokes was also an avid equestrian and when he went horseback riding one morning with one of his granddaughters, his horse disturbed a hornets' nest that sent him and the horse racing full speed into an elm tree. While he lay unconscious, his granddaughter, thrown from her horse, died from internal bleeding. Stokes abandoned the property and it went uninhabited and unattended for the next few decades.

The next owner and caretaker of Shadowbrook was also its most famous, the steel magnate Andrew Carnegie. After Carnegie fled from his native Scotland following the outbreak of World War I, he looked for a residence in America. When he visited Shadowbrook Castle and looked out at the morning mist rising from Lake Mah-keenac, surrounded by lush Green Mountains, it reminded him so much of his beloved homeland that he purchased the manor and settled onto it in 1917.

As the war ran on and expanded, Carnegie fell into despondency and died at Shadowbrook in 1919. Andrew Carnegie's widow bequeathed Shadowbrook Castle to the Order of Jesus, or the Jesuits, in 1922.

For a few decades the Jesuits flourished at Shadowbrook. Though their demise would also begin with another tragic event. In 1957, on the day before a celebration was planned to mark the 400th anniversary of the birth of the founder of the Jesuit Order, St. Ignatius Loyola, a boiler blew in the basement igniting a fire that completely destroyed the opulent mansion, while taking the lives of four young novitiates.

There was nothing left to restore, so the Jesuits started over from scratch, constructing a nondescript four-story fireproof brick building. They completed it in 1958, at a cost of $4,000.000.

They finished construction just in time to witness an unprecedented period of prosperity and liberalism sweep over America that turned many young Americans away from traditional forms of spiritual refuge and religious vocations. Declining enrollments forced the Jesuits to close the seminary in 1970.

Challenge & Triumph

Making the deal for Shadowbrook would only be half of the challenge faced by Ms. Healy and the Kripalu Yoga Fellowship.

The corporate retreat in Summit Station was, not unexpectedly, proving to be a hard sell. Try as they might, the Kripalu Yoga Fellowship could not find a buyer for it before or after they agreed to purchase Shadowbrook,

The Resignation

On New Year's Day in 1994, there would be much to celebrate at The Kripalu Center for Yoga and Health in Lenox, Massachusetts. The Center had become the largest, most successful, and fastest growing enterprise of its kind in America, and its founder and spiritual director, Yogi Amrit Desai, was esteemed as one of the most influential and innovative spiritual teachers of his generation.

Yogi Desai and The Kripalu Center earned their respective acclaim by combining an authentic and in-depth approach to yoga with an eclectic mix of modern Western techniques for promoting health, well-being and personal growth. Under the supervision of Yogi Desai, and direction of senior staff, the Kripalu Center developed a sophisticated curriculum of wellness programs and health services, complemented by a warm, welcoming staff, comfortable facilities, and first-rate modern spa facilities.

The Kripalu Center enjoyed the reputation of being a place where one could take a friend or relative and allow them to enjoy a relaxing, pampered spa retreat while you explored the most eso-teric aspects of yoga. There was no pressure exerted by Yogi Desai, or the residential staff, all of whom were devoted members of the Kripalu spiritual community, to make anyone a practitioner of Kripalu Yoga or a 'member' of the Kripalu community. The quality of the services and programs, along with the peaceful ambiance

and splendid location, gave the Kripalu Center a greater mass
appeal than any other spiritual retreat of its kind. It attracted a large
swath of middle- and upper-class Americans and Europeans, who
were intent on improving the quality of their lives, extending their
longevity, and not being pressured into anything they weren't
looking for.

Additionally, Yogi Desai and the Kripalu community had
continued to stay free of the types of public conflicts and scandals
that had overwhelmed or destroyed just about every other large
alternative spiritual community operating in the United States. The
previous decade saw Rajneeshpuram in Oregon implode, the
Siddha Yoga group in New York soiled by charges of sordid sexual
encounters, and the American self-proclaimed God-Man, Bubba
De Free John, foster a cult of personality on a private island in the
Fijis that would have made Colonel Kurtz in *Apocalypse Now* blush.

Then, in the late summer of 1994, rumors of duplicitous and
unethical conduct by Yogi Desai began to swirl through the community. The Board of Directors of The Kripalu Yoga Fellowship
felt increasing pressure from the community to meet with Yogi
Desai and talk to him about the rumors. The Board was made up of
a half-dozen senior residents, most of who had been with Kripalu
since its inception in the 1970s and had been appointed to the
Board by Yogi Desai. It was therefore not an easy or welcome task
for them to confront him with the community's concerns and
accusations.

Chief among the allegations was that Yogi Desai had been
engaged in an undisclosed, extramarital affair with the CEO of the
Kripalu Yoga Fellowship, Sandra Healey. (She'd taken a personal

leave of absence six months earlier.) And that he'd also participated in unethical business activities that allowed him to amass a personal fortune at the expense of the Fellowship and community residents.

Aids closest to Yogi Desai had been advising him for years to take the first step and admit to his actions openly and honestly in front of the community in order to diffuse what might otherwise build into an uncontrollable conflagration between him and the community. According to one of his closest personal assistants, Steven Hartman, Yogi Desai would agree, but then become distracted by other projects in order to avoid doing so. So, when the Board came to meet with him, it was not a surprise for Yogi Desai to hear what they were coming to ask him about.

As Yogi Desai listened, and for the first time acknowledged his culpability to the charges of sexual misconduct and unethical business practices, the bond of trust that had been holding the Kripalu Center and its residential community together for more than two decades was now suddenly, irrevocably, broken. The spiritual authority that had been given to Yogi Desai for the past twenty-five years was based on the shared belief that Yogi Desai did not engage in this kind of behavior, and that if he did, he would have been honest and forthright about it. If his actions betrayed those basic beliefs, and trust, than what had the spiritual community been based on all these years other than a grand shared delusion?

The Board members left the meeting crestfallen.

After taking some time to come to terms with what they just learned, the Board of Directors returned and told Yogi Desai that they wanted to meet with him again, though this time in front of the entire community. Whatever actions the Board was going to take regarding the future relationship between Kripalu and Yogi Desai were going to affect each member of the community. He agreed.

The meeting was held as soon as possible, but not before the community became abuzz with new and widening accusations – real and imagined – against their previously inviolable spiritual director.

The meeting took place in a large program room in the Center's main building. It was filled with nearly four hundred residents and staff. Yogi Desai entered and took a seat in the front of the room. The Directors then read the charges aloud and Yogi Desai once again acknowledged his complicity. The community at first fell into an awkward stunned silence.

Then a senior resident, whose ex-wife had claimed a decade earlier that she'd had a sexual encounter with Yogi Desai during a trip to India, stood up and asked Yogi Desai about that incident. Yogi Desai had denied the woman's accusations when she originally made them – causing her to be banished from the Kripalu community for lying. When Yogi Desai admitted that it had in fact taken place, it set off a vicious and vulgar harangue of insults by the ex-husband. His insults were then echoed and amplified by many other residents who suddenly felt as though years of their lives had been wasted by this corruption.

Yogi Desai found himself surrounded by an angry and threatening throng, including many new residents and temporary staff he'd never seen before, screaming and vilifying him as a conman and sexual abuser.

The Board of Directors calmed the crowd as best they could

and then demanded that Yogi Desai resign as their spiritual director
and remove himself from their property. (The Kripalu Yoga
Fellowship owned all the property and assets of the Kripalu
enterprise, except for Yogi Desai's original home and property in
Pennsylvania.) Fearing for his safety, and the legal repercussions
of his actions, Yogi Desai made his way out of the room and then
him and his family fled the property, never to return again. In less
than an hour, Yogi Desai had gone from being a respected teacher
and figure of reverence, to yet another symbol of spiritual
hypocrisy and derision. And for the first time in its history, the
Kripalu community was without a leader, or a firm direction.

EPILOGUE

To the profound credit of both Yogi Desai and the Kripalu Yoga Fellowship and Center, each has transformed since the events of 1994 that led to Yogi Desai's departure, and each has gone on to achieve a greater understanding and accomplishment of their respective missions.

Yogi Desai maintained his *sadhana* and founded the Amrit Yoga Institute in Salt Springs, Florida. He teaches less frequently and focuses his attention on practicing and revealing the deeper and more sublime aspects of yoga. For more up to date information on Yogi Desai and the Amrit Yoga institute visit AmritYoga.org.

The Kripalu Yoga Fellowship and Kripalu Center for Yoga and Health on the other hand survived a near complete financial meltdown following the departure of Yogi Amrit Desai in 1994. They are the only organization of their size to ever survive the loss of an iconic leader so closely associated with the community and enterprise. They have 'Americanized' the teaching and dissemination of yoga by becoming a professionally run non-profit educational and retreat center, and by promoting an ecumenical faculty of teachers. Yoga Journal called them the 'standard-bearers for integrity in yoga training, services and programs'.

It's written in the *Course in Miracles* that a holy place can only become Sanctified – made Sacred – when past enmities have been replaced by laughter and forgiveness.

Lets each of us take in a deep breath and on the collective exhale pray that Grace will soon bring forth the next chapter of this story – Reconciliation.

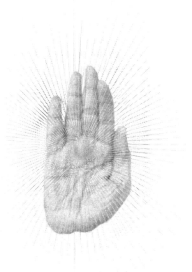

GLOSSARY

Asanas: Fundamental yoga postures.

Ashram: A spiritual retreat and/or community.

Bramacharya: A practice of moderating the senses that can include abstinence.

Charkas: Seven subtle energy centers located within the body.

Jyotirlinga: Sacred phallus representing Lord Shiva..

Kundalini: An evolutionary energy usually lying dormant in an individual until it is intentionally awakened through a process called *kundalini* yoga.

Lord Lakulish: Historical figure who formalized the practice of yoga. Also, Shrii Kripalvanandji's guru.

Linga: Phallus.

Mandir: A center for spiritual and social action.

Mantra: Repetition of sacred sounds and phrases.

Prana: Breath, or the vital life force emanating in animate beings.

Sadhana: Spiritual practices; in yoga, usually involving movement, meditation and manipulation of the breath.

Samadhi: State of bliss, peace, happiness.

Satsang: A gathering for the purpose of celebrating lightness and truthfulness.

Seva: Work, or *karma* yoga, performed as selfless service..

Shakti: A female principal of divinity in Hinduism, as well as a wellspring of creative and transformative energy in human beings.

Shaktipat-diksha: A ceremony of initiation between guru and disciple, in which highly charged and finely cultivated spiritual energy, or *shakti*, is transferred.

Shastras: Ancient Indian scriptures that outline ways to the realization of truth.

Shrii Kripalvanandji: Namesake of Kripalu Yoga; regarded in India as a saint.

Swami Shrii Ashutosh Muni: Founder of the Temple of Malav and the Kripalu Samadhi Mandir. Disciple of Shrii Kripalvanandji.

Yoga: Integration of the atomized individual with the whole self.

Yogi Amrit Desai: Founder of Kripalu Yoga and director of the Amrit Yoga Institute. Disciple of Shrii Kripalvandji.

For more information about Yogi Amrit Desai, Swami Shrii Ashutosh Muni, and the author, James Abro, visit the following websites:

AmritYoga.org

LakulishYoga.com

32BeachProductions.com

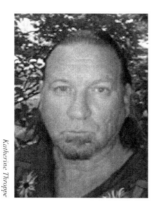

Katherine Thropp

JAMES
ABRO

James Abro began working professionally as a writer and
editor with the New York Newspaper Guild in the 1970s.
During the 1980s, he worked as Yogi Amrit Desai's book
editor on *Kripalu Yoga: Meditation in Motion*. He has
published five novels, all available for purchase on his
website, 32 Beach Productions. He has also written a memoir,
An Almost Unbearable Heartache, based on his experience
of caring for a parent with Alzheimers. Mr. Abro teaches
creative writing at a juvenile detention center, and co-facilitates
an Alzheimers Caregivers' Support Group in the town where
he lives in southern New Jersey.

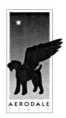

AERODALE

CPSIA information can be obtained at www.ICGtesting.com
Printed in the USA
268098BV00001B/18/P